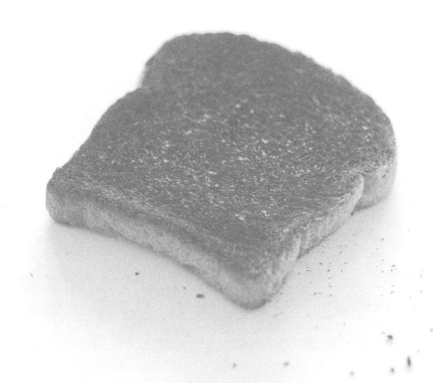

GLUTEN

is my

BITCH

GLUTEN
is my
BITCH

....

Rants, Recipes, and
RIDICULOUSNESS
for the
Gluten-Free

April Peveteaux

Stewart, Tabori & Chang | New York

Published in 2015 by Stewart, Tabori & Chang
An imprint of ABRAMS

The Library of Congress has cataloged the hardcover edition as follows:
Peveteaux, April.
  Gluten is my bitch : recipes, rants, and ridiculousness for the gluten-free / April Peveteaux.
    pages cm
  ISBN 978-1-61769-030-3 (hardback)
1. Gluten-free diet—Recipes. 2. Gluten-free foods. 3. Comfort food. I. Title.
  RM237.86.P48 2013
  641.5'63—dc23

                2013006605

Paperback ISBN: 978-1-61769-157-7

Editors: Jennifer Levesque and Camaren Subhiyah
Designer: Rachel Willey
Production Manager: Kathleen Gaffney

The text of this book was composed in Garamond, Nobel, and Freehand 575 BT.

Printed and bound in the United States
10 9 8 7 6 5 4

Stewart, Tabori & Chang books are available at special discounts when purchased in quantity for premiums and promotions as well as fund-raising or educational use. Special editions can also be created to specification. For details, contact specialsales@abramsbooks.com or the address below.

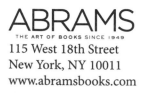

ABRAMS
THE ART OF BOOKS SINCE 1949
115 West 18th Street
New York, NY 10011
www.abramsbooks.com

For Mom.
(Sorry for all the cursing.)

Contents

Introduction

Are you perusing the "special diet" section of the bookstore right now, picking up gluten-free tomes and trying to figure out if this is the book that will be useful in your gluten-free quest (or forcible life sentence)? Let me go ahead and answer that question for you: It totally will.

I'm guessing you're looking for a little guidance, maybe some crazy delicious recipes, and a whole lot of poop jokes. You've come to the right place. But wait, there's more! I'm also here to offer you hope. Hope that someday you will feel normal again, and be able to go back to avoiding any section in the bookstore that uses the word "health" as a descriptor. Hope that even though you're giving up gluten now, you can still enjoy devil's food cake. Maybe even hope that, while you go about the business of discovering what is up with gluten-free doughnuts, a REAL doughnut might be in your future. Just wait until I tell you what medical science is up to in celiac research. Yeah, it is awesome, and I'm stoked to take you on this journey to Hopesville.

You may be wondering why I am spending my time trying to make you—the gluten intolerant—feel better about your current situation. That is a very good question, my brand-new and incredibly good-looking friend.

It was only a few years ago when I found myself in your position; wondering how I had fallen so far from being the "new fiction" browser in the store to now standing in front of the diet section looking for answers to questions about my jacked-up digestion. Sure, I was able to score some great books filled with gluten-free recipes and a few celebrity-penned tales of gluten gone wrong. Yet what I really needed was someone to tell me it was going to be all right. Not "It's going to be great! Why don't you go ahead and cut out dairy, casein, sugar, and all fun?" Instead, wondering why no one else seemed pissed off about this situation, I left the bookstore with another Swedish mystery in hand and an incredible sense of inferiority about my bad gluten-free attitude.

Just like your therapist would tell you, sometimes you have to be your own BFF. I went home and created my blog, Gluten Is My Bitch, and started talking big-time smack about gluten and the celiac disease that had suddenly appeared and taken away my villi. It helped. It really helped when I started experimenting with my deep-fat fryer, and even more so when people seemed to enjoy learning how to make gluten-free cakes, pies, and cookies as much as I enjoyed eating the creations. And that's why this book is sitting in your hands. The gluten-free people want to eat cake. The fact is, more and more people are going gluten-free and all of them aren't into mixing twenty-eight flours to make the perfect soufflé, or chanting "I'm Grateful" while they dine out. Those people need some Gluten Is My Bitch in their lives. Just like you do!

Let's bring it down for just a minute. Here's the thing about going gluten-free, whether you've been given a celiac disease diagnosis or just know you feel better when you're not enjoying cinnamon rolls for breakfast, flatbread pizza for lunch, and a pile of spaghetti Bolognese for dinner: It's fucking hard. I won't sugarcoat that for you, so if you're looking for a book to cheerlead you all the way to Vegantown, maybe look up and to your left. (Note: I do have some amazing gluten-free and vegan recipes inside these pages, 'cuz I'm all-inclusive like that.) Smiling through the pain of watching your friends enjoy unlimited breadsticks while your plate sits empty does not change the intensity of our shared gluten-free torment. Let's own that pain and complain about it until we're asked to leave the party. It's not all about wallowing in self-pity, though plenty of that is certainly in order. You are giving up chocolate croissants, after all.

Gluten Is My Bitch: Rants, Recipes, and Ridiculousness for the Gluten-Free will try a little bit to make you see the bright side, but if you don't want to, I won't dismiss you as "difficult" and will instead take you out for tequila shots (naturally gluten-free, y'all!) and tacos. I'll also tell you plenty of off-color jokes on the way to conquering your gluten-free diet, and hold your hair when you throw up. We are a unique people who cannot enjoy the best of what the bakery has to offer any longer, and so therefore we deserve special treatment, yet no one really wants to give it to us. But I will. In fact, I am! I'm ready to pamper you and poke with a stick anyone who dares get in my way. That's just the kind of gal I am.

Perhaps, before delving into *Gluten Is My Bitch*, you would like to see some credentials. How about I ask the same of you? As someone who knows how to use the hell out of Google, I will now diagnosis you based on symptoms and Internet searches. Those of you who discover through my incredibly nonprofessional quiz that you are, indeed, gluten intolerant are welcome. The rest of you are welcome too, but you should really see someone about that gout. Ready? Answer me this:

1. When I wake up in the morning:

a) I have to throw up.
b) My sheets feel like they are slicing my big toe into a million pieces.
c) My energy is at its highest and I jump out of bed, excited to begin a new day.
d) I'm still tired.

2. After lunch, I usually:

a) Feel good for the first time all day, at least until I get hungry half an hour later.
b) Wonder what's up with my throbbing big toe.
c) Hit the gym—it's the best time to take advantage of my post-lunch energy boost.
d) Poop my pants.

3. The last thing I think about before I go to sleep is:

a) Is it too early to have breakfast?
b) Is it okay to wear ski boots to bed, on account of this pain in my toe that is aggravated by my sheets?
c) I had the most amazing day and I feel GREAT!
d) Wow, I sure am . . . zzzzzzzz . . .

If you answered *a* on every question: Congratulations, you're pregnant!
If you answered *b* on every question: Damn, son, you've got the gout.
If you answered *c* on every question: I fucking hate you.
If you answered *d* on every question: Yep, you've got a gluten problem.

For all of you "d" people, come join me in the gluten-free world as I continue to make new discoveries, with much emphasis on the ridiculousness of our shared bread-free situation. Really, it's OK in here. I mean, not as OK as eating brioche every day for breakfast, but it'll do. Welcome.

Chapter One

WHAT TO DO WHEN YOU'RE

Crapping Your Pants

Hello there! If you picked up this book because you're crapping your pants, I have to say you've come to the right place. So pull up your bowl and squat because I can fill you in on what funny things are happening to your body. Almost as uncomfortable as "the talk" we're going to go through your digestive system and work out what this crazy problem actually is, or is not. Most likely you're blaming gluten right about now because, come on, *it's the worst*. Do you have the autoimmune disorder celiac disease? (Note: If you're European, it's coeliac or the very cutely named, "sprue." Lucky Europeans.) Do you have a wheat allergy? Or are you one of those illusive "gluten intolerants"? Maybe you've decided it's about time you tried that paleo diet all the kids are talking about. Whatever your gluten situation, you're probably here because there is pooping, or perhaps, retching involved. If you're super lucky you'll also have a little itchiness, a bit of achiness, or all around crankiness. Which means it's time to start making some incredibly painful and permanent choices about the most important thing in your life, which is, of course, food. If you thought it was something else, perhaps you should look at a different book, like say, *The Secret*. But if you're here to learn about your weird physical ailments, read on my disgusting friends.

So, what seems to be the problem? Check one:

 I am bloated, gassy, and no fun to be around.

 I have a rash that won't go away. No, it's not syphilis. Stop looking at me that way.

 I'm so tired I've given up on the disco nap and just take a pre-bedtime nap.

 I'm pretty sure I'm allergic to turkey, rather than the delicious sourdough it is served upon. Stupid turkey.

 Between the brain fog and the creaky joints, I've turned into that old guy who screams at empty chairs.

 I'm losing a scary amount of weight, and it's really not awesome anymore.

Or perhaps, you, like me, had violent diarrhea for three months straight, wound up in the hospital, and finally decided to take control of your digestive situation.

We are a fun bunch, are we not?

No matter what kind of sickness has taken hold of you, let's blame gluten. If you want or need to get gluten out of your diet, bravo! Kick that nasty gluten to the curb, I say. Pretend it's an unwanted cat (which I'm also allergic to, so *no problem*), or that one ex-partner who is such a mistake you still cringe when you think about being seen with him/her. What were you thinking? Really?

But before you totally and completely ban wheat, barley, rye, and the odd man out—triticale—you should consider the following:

- Maybe it really *is* the turkey.

- Perhaps you just have pinworms. In which case, whew! (And please never sleep over at my house.)

- I hate to even bring this up, but it could be the dairy.

- You've been watching too much *Grey's Anatomy* and are self-diagnosing without a medical degree or improv classes.

- You don't realize beer and cake both have gluten.

After contemplating all of the above, and more, you still may want to cut gluten out of your diet. I'm not here to discourage you but simply to make sure you totally get that gluten tastes awesome, and you should seriously consider what your life would look like without gluten. (It will look cake-less and beer-less, FYI.) But if you've been diagnosed with celiac disease, or you're one of the twenty million Americans stricken with gluten sensitivity, it's time to kick some gluten ass—and read this book.

Not sure if gluten-free is for you? Perhaps gluten simply causes you some discomfort, but you've never been diagnosed. Then eff that gluten! Get it out of your system, ban it from your cupboard, and kick it out, with my help. The fact is, gluten sensitivity can be damn tricky to diagnosis, even though your symptoms are the same—or worse—than those of your friend who looks totally legit, what with her celiac disease diagnosis. Don't let anyone tell you it's all in your head because even if it *is* all in your head, it's still coming out of your rear parts. If something is making you sick, stay away from it, no matter how tempting. That includes beer and cake, dammit.

Listen, some people will make you feel bad for wanting to disrespect gluten. After all, bread is the staff of life and all that. Some of us with celiac disease might think you're just trying to be trendy, and you could possibly hurt our reputation. Personally, my reputation is already shot the minute I walk into a restaurant and identify myself as having special needs—so I'm cool with all that. If you don't want gluten in your life, send it packing. Honestly, no matter which way you come to gluten-free, I will not judge. I will, however, feel super stoked to have a meal with you so I won't be the only weirdo at the table.

For those of you who have been suffering in silence, or suffering loudly and obnoxiously; or those who have suddenly found yourselves getting sick every time you grab lunch at the fried-chicken palace; or even those who just like reading scatological nonfiction—welcome. No matter why you're here, I'm going to help you out and off the pot. Or at least, help you laugh while you're on the pot. Which is really how all great works should be measured: Does it keep me entertained whilst on the pot?

I realize that some of you are incredibly angry right now. Those of you with small children with celiac are ready to punch a doctor then cry yourself to sleep for the next six months. It's true that this is a crappy situation. But we can get through it together, if only we make fun of it and learn how to eat Buffalo wings again without getting violently ill. That's a laudable goal, for us gluten-haters. You may not feel like you're ready to laugh yet, but I say you are. Since I am the boss of this book, you must obey or have a time out while you think about your actions.

Ready? Even if—out of a strict sense of duty or gravity—you insist on keeping your laugh lines perfectly straight throughout the reading of this guide, I'm still going to help you conquer that devil gluten. Exorcise it from your life, and your gut, and replace it with much better options, as well as lots of confidence when you head out to dinner. No more contemplating adult diapers or resorting to wearing your old granny panties on dinner dates. This no-bullshit guide is going to allow you to live loud, proud, and gluten-free.

Who the Heck Are You?

You may be thinking, "Hey, April has celiac disease. Why is she so dang happy? How does she stay so Zen when she can't order off the menu anymore without harassing the entire waitstaff and the chef? How is it she can laugh about this whole gluten-free diet suckage when it does, indeed, suck so much?"

Here's the thing. First of all, it's an angry laugh. Plus, I've had a little bit of time to work through my deprivation issues and gluten challenges. I was once like you: just waking up from anesthesia and finding out that "Waffle Wednesdays" are now a thing of the past. Sure I was angry, peeved, and petulant. But then I realized how to be totally, 100 percent OK with cutting gluten out of my diet. It's absolutely no problem to go gluten-free as long *as everyone else in the entire world does it too.*

Since it seems like this is the way people are going, well, we celiacs have really won this war, don't you think? Approximately three million Americans have celiac disease, and probably two million poor saps are going around without knowing they are part of the club: pooping, crying, and wondering what the heck is going on with their digestive system. *There are twenty million of us who are gluten intolerant.* That's a huge amount of people clamoring for gluten-free goods! There are athletes, celebrities, and crazy people, all demanding gluten-free food be shoved into their gullets. Which is actually great for us celiac types because now we can walk into French Laundry and get gluten-free bread. Wendy's offers a gluten-free menu—some of the gluten-free foodstuffs even qualify as "value." We've won! Now, don't you feel better? No? Darn it; are you still bloated and irritable? OK, then, let's get real.

How Do You Know If Gluten Is Really the One?

Just like your latest Internet date, it can be difficult to figure out if gluten is the one you should never, ever see or talk to or breathe upon again. The fact of the matter is that celiacs take an average of ten years[1] to get diagnosed. So you may be going around crapping your pants for a very long time and hearing doctors tell you that it's all in your head or that you're just "stressed." Of course you're stressed: YOU'RE CRAPPING YOUR PANTS. Because there is no test for the gluten intolerant, you guys just have to figure this business out for yourselves. With the average diagnosis of celiac disease taking so

---

1 Six to ten years is the average time a person waits to be correctly diagnosed. (Source: Daniel Leffler, M.D., M.S., The Celiac Center at Beth Israel Deaconness Medical Center.)

damn long, and no quick way to alert the gluten sensitive, you can understand why so many celiacs and intolerants are kind of downers. That's ten years (or more!) of doctors telling you to go home and eat more yogurt. I can't even imagine what it would be like to be sick for ten years with no diagnosis. Which is why I consider myself extremely lucky to have gotten violently ill continuously until I had to admit that the only option was to have someone knock me out and shove something up my butt and down my throat.

Which brings us to how you know you have celiac disease. Celiac disease can be diagnosed in a few different ways, but the proof is in the villi. You know, those hairy-looking things in your small intestine that suck up all the vitamins and nutrients your body needs to function? If you have the auto-immune disease of celiac, you can say good-bye to those cute little villi. In fact, mine were completely gone. Or as my gastroenterologist said, "It looks like someone took an axe to your villi." Nice violent imagery there, but I'm pretty sure he felt he had to get brutal with someone who let her body become completely worn down without picking up the phone to call a doctor until she wound up in the emergency room. The good news is, if your villi are gone, your doctor can tell you with confidence that you have celiac disease.[2]

The bad news is, your villi are gone and you have celiac disease. But yet again, the good news is, I'm totally going to help you figure out how to live without gluten. Hooray, me! Hooray, you! Boo, gluten!

If you went straight for the endoscopy and learned about your villi situation, you're good, as well as a total badass. But if you want to start slowly, perhaps your first step toward celiac diagnosis will involve a tissue transglutaminase antibody test, which is also known as the tTG test. This test shows if you have antibodies that are consistent with celiac disease. Maybe your blood test came back positive for celiac disease. Hey, mine did too! But the blood test also came back positive for Crohn's disease, which is a heck of a lot scarier than celiac. (If you're Crohn's and gluten-free, welcome! I love your kind and have nothing but respect for those of you who aren't just, like, "Fuck it,

---

2 I am so totally not a doctor. I just write books about disgusting medical conditions. Please consult your doctor for a proper diagnosis.

take out my intestines so I can eat biscuits and gravy." Hell, I have respect for those of you who *do* say that. Mad respect.) So this is why the biopsy via endoscopy is always a fantastic idea in order to get an accurate diagnosis.

If you haven't been offered this biopsy option, you need to get serious with your doctor. Although I was rushed into the endoscopy and colonoscopy option, I've heard horror stories of people who were ignored by their doctors, never taken seriously when they complained of aches, pains, rashes, diarrhea, vomiting, and all-around unwellness. If you find yourself in a doctor's office with an unresponsive physician, you've got to be loud and *demand* a diagnosis. Celiac is no joke, nor is any food allergy or intolerance. They may be easy to make fun of, but if you don't have celiac under control, it can be

Craziest Things I've Said While Suffering a Gluten Attack

1. Here, take this Ziploc bag of poop to the emergency room and have them analyze it.

2. I know I said before that if I died, I didn't want you to re-marry, but now that I think it's going to happen, do what you've got to do.

3. I really don't think it was the gluten.

4. Can you please go get me a skinny vanilla latte?

5. I'm fine.

life threatening. I'll get into all the awesome diseases undiagnosed celiac can bring on later, but right now we're only talking about pleasant things. Like how I found out I could no longer visit The Grilled Cheese Truck when it was so thoughtfully parked in the Frosted Cupcakery parking lot.

About Me and My Disgusting, Disgusting Body

Not surprisingly, my digestive issues began shortly after I moved to Los Angeles. Also not surprisingly, I blamed everything on my cross-country move as I left behind my beloved Brooklyn, along with all of my street cred. But I had a family now, and one must do what's best for the children, and that meant moving somewhere with perfect weather and employment opportunities for the man who makes the real money in our household—my husband. After all, I'm just a writer, and we all know how the Internet has ruined all of our chances of ever making money again. So thank you for buying this book and allowing me to purchase my very expensive gluten-free saltines. You may also need to get a second job (or write a book, 'cuz you know, it's *super easy*) in order to afford all of those new gluten-free foods. But we'll explore that later, when I take you on a journey through the supermarket.

Back to the pooping and Los Angeles. Like I said, I was ripped from Brooklyn and plopped down in Southern California, where I worked from home and shuttled my kids around to day care and preschool. Every now and then I would find myself in debilitating pain and hanging out on the pot all day. As someone who had previously eaten Mexican food and barbecue at every single meal, I was shocked at my sudden delicate constitution. Yet I ignored it. Or rather, tried to work around it.

And everything would have been fine had it not been for my husband and his love of not having a heart attack in his thirties. Suddenly the man I married had the genius idea that we should try to go vegetarian for a month. Give it the old college try, since hey, we'd done it for an entire week a few years ago and that worked out *not at all* well. Why not go for an entire month of getting creative in the kitchen, which also translates to buying things in packages and reheating? Here's how it all went horribly wrong: You know what vegetarians eat, right? Gluten. Those people eat tons and tons of gluten. You've got your seitan and your pasta, your couscous, and lots of grilled cheese sandwiches. And this is why I can blame my celiac disease on vegetarianism and/or my husband.

Instead of feeling light and airy and super smug about not eating meat, I instead found myself in a constant state of beshatting. Still, I was blaming my move, my stressful job, and the lack of insulation in our rental home (seriously, California, get it together). For a moment I even blamed my best friend, dairy. But that didn't last long because I really couldn't stay mad at dairy. Can anyone? In hindsight, I'd had a few severe bouts of stomach distress in the previous year, and I was convinced that I had developed arthritis at a very young age. Then there was that whole winter in New York when I thought the cold was responsible for my dry, flaky skin, yet it did not change even when I visited Texas, the land of humidity and the burrito. So even though the vegetarianism put me totally over the edge, the celiac symptoms had been slowly sneaking up, ready to attack as soon as they had a great reason. That great reason was pasta every day for a month.

It wasn't until I wound up in the emergency room because I was pretty sure my stomach was about to rip out of my body, and I couldn't even breathe through the pain, that I finally took some advice from the ER doc. Two months later I walked into my fantastic GI doctor's office (I know! How stubborn am I?) and was quickly scheduled for an endoscopy and colonoscopy.

If you've never had the joy of a procedure that requires you empty out your entire insides before even stepping inside the doctor's office, you are missing out on a serious good time. Yet here's how sick I had been up until that point: When it was my turn to drink that battery acid that clears out your entire digestive system for, like, two days, it didn't even faze me. Yep, my daily living with explosive diarrhea was much worse than the colon blow most people avoid even at the cost of dying from cancer. I remember coming out of the bathroom at midnight after about sixteen hours of the pre-colonoscopy regimen and saying to my husband, "Huh, that's not so bad."

What's also not so bad is the entire procedure if you have the proper insurance. I highly recommend you do make sure the procedure is covered before you wander into the hospital because you want to be completely knocked out for an endoscopy and/or colonoscopy. Trust me on this one. Go sell a few pieces of jewelry to cover the general anesthesia if it's not covered. *Because someone is going to shove a tube with a camera down your throat and up your rectum.* You do NOT want to be awake for that. Also, you don't want to hear what everyone is saying about you in the procedure room as they get an intimate look at areas of your body that process food into waste.

When I finally did wake up, none the wiser about the violations that had just taken place, I learned that I did indeed have celiac disease. Shockingly, this was a relief that perhaps you too can relate to when you finally figure out what the heck is going on with your body. Because my first thought was *Thank god it wasn't cancer or Crohn's*. Sorry, Crohn's people, again—I wish I could wave a magic wand over your insides. But then I had some even more urgent thoughts, ones that you may have as well.

Questions you may have, and should totally ask, when you wake up from the anesthesia:

- Can I eat cake?

- Can I eat cupcakes?

- What about those mini cupcakes?

- Not even on my birthday?

- Who the hell do you think you are?

- Is that even a *real* college? Or did you get that degree from a Cracker Jack box?

- Can I eat Cracker Jack?

- Did you leave your head up my butt while you were in there?

- Are you sure?

- Then you won't mind if I shove something up *your* butt?

Hopefully your GI doc will be as chill as mine and won't threaten to go back in while you're awake and "can really feel it."

It's shocking to discover you can't eat something that is basically everywhere and in everything you want to eat. Especially shocking because I honestly don't know if I had even *heard* of gluten at that point. Of course I was about to get intimately acquainted with that toxic beast. By intimately acquainted, I mean stalking it and bad-mouthing it to anyone who would listen, followed by lots of crying because I missed that awful gluten.

It's true that this whole procedure of the emptying of your bowels, being

By the Numbers

Approximately three million Americans have been diagnosed with celiac disease, and the working theory is that another two million are going around eating gluten willy-nilly and getting sick, without a diagnosis. There are twenty million Americans who are gluten intolerant, poor things. So there are quite a few of us here in the U.S.A. trying to get rid of the gluten in our lives. To help you get a visual of how many of us are out there shopping, talking back to waiters, and being generally aggressive about our food, here's how the gluten-free stack up to other populations in America.

There are more people who can't eat the devil gluten than:

- Juggalos at the annual Insane Clown Posse Gathering
- Voted for Ross Perot for president of the United States in 1992
- Breastfeed their baby until the age of one year. Not that it's any of your damn business.
- Know all the words to "Free Bird"

There are fewer people who can't eat the devil gluten than:

- Are "Single" on Facebook
- Ryan Gosling fans
- Voted for Michael Dukakis for president of the United States (who knew?)
- Have sung the chorus of "Sweet Caroline" loudly, while drunk, at a bar
- Have forgotten about singing "Sweet Caroline" loudly, while drunk, somewhere that they can't quite recall

knocked out, and having things shoved inside of you is unpleasant, but it is a necessary step to make sure you have celiac disease. Then you can rest easy knowing that you can never eat gluten again for the rest of your life. And that's how the procedure goes, unless you're one of those people who have celiac disease but never have any gastrointestinal problems. Oh, hell, you didn't realize that was a thing, did you?

What to Do If You're NOT Crapping Your Pants

Let's talk about *that* whackness. For some celiacs, or some people who simply react badly to consuming gluten, it's not the pooping that drives them to diagnosis. There are a whole host of non-gastrointestinal symptoms that are related to celiac disease, including dermatitis herpetiformis. After you say that five times fast, you're going to have an itchy, red rash to scratch, thanks to gluten. Even though you're not having diarrhea, constipation, or vomiting, if you have celiac you're just as unable to absorb the necessary nutrients and can still face all those fun diseases like cancer or osteoporosis if you do not get diagnosed and get on that gluten-free diet. Other symptoms of celiac that are non-gastro-related include:

- Depression
- Brain fog
- Anemia
- Joint pain/Arthritis
- Muscle cramps
- Mouth sores
- Acid reflux
- Dental and bone disorders
- Neuropathy (tingling in your extremities)
- Exhaustion and weakness
- Stunted growth

- Weight loss

- Fertility problems and miscarriage

- Anxiety (Aren't you getting anxious just reading this list?)

- Migraines

- Acne

- Eczema

So what I'm trying to say is, having celiac disease as well as gluten sensitivity is an amazing time, and you'll always be the life of the party.

Why Me?

If you're as self-indulgent as I am, you may be wondering why in the name of all things holy you wound up with this autoimmune disorder or allergic reaction, or intolerance, or whatever the heck it is that's going down in your intestines. Although historically the medical community believed this was a white person's disease—specifically people from the UK and wherever they colonized (which is a lot of places, *amiright?*)—celiac and gluten sensitivity has now been discovered on every continent. Which means we're not alone. Sure, you may be Irish, but you don't *have* to be to have sprue. Also, it's possible to have the genetic markers for the sprue but no symptoms for a very long time. Which is what happened to me, until one fateful day with a frozen pizza.

One theory I floated to my gastroenterologist and my nutritionist—that they both seemed to be on board with—was that my recent food poisoning had something to do with my current condition. Although no one was willing to go on record and confirm, I've heard anecdotes about food poisoning being the beginning of the end of a gluten-filled diet. In fact, if you want me to get all celebrity on you, *The View* cohost and token Republican, Elisabeth Hasselbeck, and I both have celiac, and we both had a major incident with food poisoning prior to getting all sick in our pants. See? Two ladies, one common thread.

Apparently we are not alone in that because there is a brand-spanking-new study that has shown a connection between gastroenteritis and celiac disease[3] wherein patients experience a bacterial intestinal infection twenty-four months prior to experiencing symptoms of celiac disease. Although more studies need to be done, this is the beginning of research that totally backs me up in my theory that had I skipped a poison pizza, I'd still be enjoying doughnuts. Because it is clear to me that I was eating the hell out of gluten, and never had any physical ailment as a result, before I wound up in the hospital with severe food poisoning. I also was incredibly lucky to have had two very healthy pregnancies before this particular hammer came down upon me, which is challenging for a celiac woman who wishes to reproduce. So there.

In the summer of 2009, right after my son was born, I was enjoying a frozen pizza with not one, not two, but THREE meats atop its crust. Within about an hour I was emptying my bowels and my stomach with such severity that I began to resemble an opiate addict detoxing on *Celebrity Rehab with Dr. Drew*. Which may be why the fine people at the Brooklyn emergency room I found myself in did not take me seriously and I almost died. My general practitioner determined that it was E. coli, or salmonella, or some kind of serious poisoning that came from meat. Since the only meat I had eaten (or the only three meats I had eaten) in several days had come from that nasty-ass pizza, I wrote a letter to Stouffer's. I got a check for $20 and some coupons for more Lean Cuisine products, and apparently the beginning of my celiac disease symptoms. A note to Lean Cuisine: If someone gets violently ill on your product, a coupon to eat it again may not sway him or her. Maybe.

I'm not sure whether to curse the day Mr. and Mrs. Stouffer conceived baby Stouffer, who then tried his hand at a leaner cuisine, or to thank them for helping me identify a potentially life-threatening disease. I'm going with cursing because this was most likely the trigger for my gastrointestinal symptoms, which just might have been dormant and thus allowing me to enjoy wedding cake instead of sitting in the back, cursing love. At the same time, I come from a family fairly riddled with autoimmune disorders, and celiac

---

3 Reuters Health, July 4, 2012.

apparently is mine. Woo-hoo! Yet with any autoimmune disease, the whys and hows are incredibly shady. This is why anyone with a weird autoimmune thing will experience intense frustration with getting a diagnosis and trying to find a treatment. But luckily for those of us getting diagnosed now, there is much more awareness and much less "This is so totally in your head. Take a Valium and call me next year." Not that I wouldn't mind a Valium when I'm at yet another school function that starts directly after work when I'm at maximum starvation and that serves only pasta and bread.

If you're one of those people who have gluten sensitivity, it's possible it took even longer for you to figure out what was bugging you. I've known people who were so sick they began the elimination diet in earnest, only to drop it after four days of eating air. I also wonder how many doctors who have prescribed the elimination diet have actually done it themselves because that is one ridiculous thing to do to yourself. If you've never been on the elimination diet, consider yourself lucky. Here's what you're not allowed to eat, in pursuit of what food is making your body miserable: dairy, eggs, gluten, corn, sulfites (wine! Ahhhhhh!), soy, citrus fruits, caffeine (again, ahhhhhhh!), and all processed foods. So enjoy that hunk of grass-fed meat for a few weeks 'cause that's all you can have. If you came to your gluten intolerance diagnosis in this manner, I salute you while thanking god for my violent illness so I didn't have to do this crazy diet.

There IS a super-duper silver lining to all of this (or so I keep telling myself): You have a disease that's 100 percent reversible if you do one thing. Yes, that one thing is to never eat gluten again for the rest of your life. And while that may suck, it's a heck of a lot better than having to medicate, receive blood transfusions, or organ transplants. Don't you feel better already? No?

Then come with me and figure out how you can turn that intolerant, allergic, or celiac frown upside down! It's time to bust up some gluten and dive into the gluten-free pool of deliciousness. No, I'm not kidding. You can have deliciousness without gluten. I swear on my mother's muffin pan.

Chapter Two

SO YOU CAN'T EAT

Gluten

ANYMORE

You may be sitting at home right now with a steak and a head of broccoli. If so, good for you! *That's totally gluten-free.* Don't let anyone tell you it's weird to sit around with your food in your lap, massaging it gently and pondering life. You're off to a fantastic start. Although steak and broccoli do make a perfectly acceptable meal, at some point you're going to want to branch out. That means you're going to have to go grocery shopping. You're also going to have to take out a loan to buy lots of gluten-free substitutes. Because gluten-free food costs more to produce, what with its fancy clean machinery, low demand, weird grains, and with no gluten dripping all over the place. That cost, of course, is passed on to you. I'm just telling you because I don't want you to get sticker shock the first time you pick up your gluten-free crackers and gluten-free beer for the holiday weekend. Because nothing says "party" like crackers and beer! You are welcome. And here's where I give you the good news: Gluten-free food for the sick is tax deductible under medical expenses. What? That's right, gluten-free food is like your medicine now, people. So write that shizzle off.[4]

---

4 Talk to your accountant to make this legal, not some lady writing a book with a curse word in the title.

But before you go crazy like I did, don't race to your local health food store and buy up everything with a GF label and go home and make amaranth doughnuts, sorghum doughnuts, rice doughnuts, and gluten-free potato chip doughnuts. Stop and assess your new lifestyle. Yes, it is a lifestyle even if it's been forcibly imposed. Maybe you only need two varieties of gluten-free chocolate chip cookie dough. And probably one gluten-free brownie mix will do it for you. Oh, hell, what do I care? *Go crazy in the gluten-free aisle* (or shelf, as your store may not be with it just yet). It will be cathartic. Stock those cabinets with buckwheat noodles and gluten-free scone mix. Try your hand at recreating Chelsea Clinton's gluten-free wedding cake! Why not? But just in case you don't want to spend your entire paycheck on gluten-free options that you wind up throwing in the trash, maybe keep reading.

Your new diet food can be categorized in two ways: the naturally gluten-free and the not-at-all naturally gluten-free but it is now thanks to science. I feel the urge to tell you that naturally gluten-free food is going to be the better choice. However, you're going to want some of that not-natural stuff as well *because it's delicious.* Not as delicious as that Twix bar you can no longer have, but food companies are making great strides, and I honestly expect the Twix people to present me with a delicious gluten-free version any day now. I'm waiting.

Here's how it all breaks down.

Naturally Gluten-Free Foods That Are Your New Best Friends

You'll be shocked at all the foods that contain the devil gluten. But since you probably never paid one second of attention to gluten before, you might be just as shocked at the quantity of foods that do not naturally contain gluten. These foods are your very best friends. You don't have to specially prepare them or mix them while crying because the xanthan gum is making your fingers all weirdly slippery. (Oh, you'll find out all about xanthan gum, don't you worry.) You can just pick them off a tree, slice them off an animal, or milk them from a cow, and you're good to go. That's why that broccoli-and-steak dinner was such a great idea. Good job for thinking of that!

Just like all those people who write books with rules on how to eat healthy and avoid the grocery store glut, if you stick to the aisles around the sides of the store you'll probably be safe. I mean, not totally safe. There's sausage out there, after all. But here are the safest, and chilliest, sections of the grocery store to get your gluten-free eat on:

- Butcher/Fish counter
- Produce (that's fruits and vegetables for you former fast-food devotees)
- Dairy

Bring your sweater.

Meat Is the Word

Meat and fish, in its natural form, is totally gluten-free. Yes, even grass-fed beef. (That was an actual question Ɨ someone had—don't make fun.) Please note that packaged meat is not in its natural form. Meat with "natural flavors" is not at all natural, and you must find out what those flavors are made of because a lot of times those flavors are made out of gluten. The good news is, if you're shopping for cuts of meat with the help of your butcher, so long as no one has slathered a marinade or bread crumbs all over it, you're safe to buy out the entire store and go home and eat it. That's right, I just gave you permission to go on a meat gorge. Go crazy! Oh, except for that one super-delicious meat.

The delicious, yet deadly, sausage I mentioned earlier, for example. You don't have to give up sausage completely (thank you, gluten-loving Jesus!), you just have to do one of two things: Buy gluten-free sausage or make sausage at home yourself. Sometimes the latter is actually easier because people love to fill up tube meats with other business that, although delicious, will make the gluten intolerant keel over. Even if you're buying sausage from your friendly neighborhood butcher, he might be using a wheat-based casing around that pure sausage meat. Ahem, I said "pure." Obviously the same goes for hot dogs. Do not eat a dog until you've checked its credentials. This is good advice in any situation. For both sausage and hot dogs, I have found that Applegate does a damn good job of keeping the mixed meat gluten-free. It's also organic and anti-antibiotic, which is only helpful to those of us with issues. Yes, I just strongly implied that you should go organic. Don't hate.

Why Go Organic?

I'm not here to tell you that you can only put organic quinoa in your body from now on (though someone will tell you that, you can bet on it), but I will say this—the less junk in your food, the less likely you'll wind up on the bowl. Organic produce, dairy, meat, even organic processed food is simply better for your body's digestive system. The less crap up in there, the better. You're sensitive now; act like it.

Organic means no synthetic pesticides used on your food, no human sewage fertilizer used (ewwwww! Now you'll *never* eat nonorganic, right?), no antibiotics used in animals, and strict separation of organic and nonorganic crops grown with the help of chemicals. It is hoped all organic products will begin to also be labeled as non-GMO foods, and GMO foods will soon be labeled as such. That's genetically modified organisms, for those of you keeping score at home, and that means food that has been messed with, and not for the better. Say it with me: "No more GMOs! No more GMOs!" Ready to storm the castle? Let's have some organic gluten-free chocolate first, shall we?

To recap: Spend the extra and go organic, just so you know you're not getting poisonous compounds along with your grapes. Your beat-up stomach will thank you. Unless you can't find it, you can't afford it, or some other reason like "Seriously? Why are you telling me what to do? You promised not to tell me what to do!" It's OK, you do what you've got to do to stay gluten-free and able to pay your rent. I'm just saying organic is where it's at.

Produce

It's a fact that you can eat as many greens as you'd like and ingest zero gluten. That also goes for oranges, reds, purples, and whatever other colors you find in your fruits and vegetables. In their original form, fruits and vegetables are gluten-free. Just don't add any gluten to that business, and you'll be good. Sadly, this also means "pie." You cannot add pie to your fruit and still be eating gluten-free. Unless, of course, you use one of my gluten-free pie recipes! I *told* you this book was going to be good.

Really, any produce is great for you, and of course, most of it should be organic. See page 33 for organic diatribe. If it's not available to you, or it's just too dang expensive, at the very least buy these "dirty dozen[5]" foods in the organic section. These are the fruits and vegetables most easily contaminated by pesticides:

- Peaches
- Apples
- Sweet bell peppers
- Nectarines, imported
- Strawberries
- Celery
- Lettuce
- Potatoes
- Grapes
- Spinach
- Cucumbers
- Blueberries

---

5 Environmental Working Group

I don't mean to harp on the organic thing. For those of you who read the study out of Stanford that said organic is not more healthy than nonorganic, remember that I'm talking to you—the people with food issues. It's not that you're looking for a healthier apple with more vitamins; instead you're looking for an apple that hasn't been sprayed with chemicals or crossbred with an almond that could wreak havoc on your sensitive gut. I just want to make sure you know what's up with your groceries. I'm also not saying one can live on produce alone, but if you're like, "Oh my god! Everything has gluten! I can't eat one damn thing!!!" remember: produce. It's your gluten-free buddy. You can always roll that orange in sugar and/or beef if you're really feeling panicked. In fact, that's one of my recipes! (*Editor's note: It's totally not one of her recipes; that is disgusting.*)

Cheese, Beautiful Cheese

I worked hard to earn the nickname "The Dairy Queen," which is why it was such a shock to me when I heard that oftentimes gluten and dairy problems go together. I was even more shocked when someone implied that perhaps it would be a great idea for me to go dairy-free. And imagine how shocked he was when he wound up in a headlock, between my armpit and my bosom.

I love dairy. I love cheese, butter, and cheesy-butter. I think milkshakes are the nectar of the gods, and I wouldn't kick a fro-yo out of my bed. For those of us who are on restricted diets, it's these other comfort foods that will get us through. Mine happens to be dairy. You'll find your own, but if you're searching: May I suggest dairy? If you must be dairy-free, allow me to offer my most sincere condolences and suggest you skip right over to the next section. Also, check out my vegan recipes because they are also delicious. No, I'm not kidding.

If you're lucky like me, however, you'll get much enjoyment by bulking up on almost every single dairy product. Notice I said almost. Although a recent report came out saying blue cheese is now OK for the gluten intolerant, I've heard many murmurings that the opposite is true. Apparently there's this thing about the bread mold that makes the blue business all up on the cheese. Bread that has gluten. Gluten that hates you. I'm sure by the time this book winds up on shelves and somewhere in cyberspace, someone will have tossed out another opinion on the elusive blue cheese. So unless you think you'll die without it, skip it until you hear otherwise. Remember, there's always Gouda. Here's where I remind you again—go organic and antibiotic free. You really, really, really don't want weird stuff in your dairy because it travels through your body and turns right into man boobs.

I would be remiss in not pointing out that not all foods found in the dairy section of your grocery are created equal. Of course cheese, yogurt, milk, and butter in the purest form are all naturally gluten-free. But dairy is so damn good, people love to get in there and muck it up. That's because they're just jealous. You've seen that yogurt with the M&Ms and granola? If only they'd stopped at the M&Ms, you'd be safe. Granola, however, is a killer. Every processed food—even those made from beloved dairy—must be scrutinized. It was perhaps one of the saddest days of my life when my go-to spinach-artichoke dip was marked off my faves list due to the words "Made in a facility that processes wheat." Sure, it's possible that wheat-processing machine never touched my dip, but who knows? Not me. At least, not until I wound up bent over the toilet bowl.

And that's the thing about going gluten-free: Some of us are more sensitive than others. If you happen to have celiac disease, or just happen to be really, really, sensitive, you can't even eat gluten-free food that has interacted with gluten. By interacting I mean made in the same mixer, factory, or even kitchen. Which brings us to the conversation I've been dreading: the cross-contamination discussion.

Cross-Contamination: Buyer Beware

Whether you're dining out, dining in, grocery shopping, or Dumpster diving, you've got to take notice of where your gluten-free food has been. You are now a gluten-free food stalker, and you must embrace this creepy fact.

Sometimes identifying gluten-free contaminated food is as obvious as trying to pry that Brie off a baguette, other times it's totally unclear and no, you do not understand why you cannot have that gluten-free pizza that was made on the same surface as a gluten-filled pizza. Especially since not one single ingredient is gluten. The thing is, gluten is sticky. If you put a croissant down on a plate, some croissant-y gluten will stick to it. So don't even think about licking that plate in hopes of tasting croissant again. Trust me on that one.

The bummer of the situation is, if you pick up a food that has also been processed on the same machinery—or sometimes in the same facility—as wheat, you can get glutened. That's why the little gluten-free symbol on packaged foods is so hard to get. That business has to be clean. This is also why if you make a (gluten-free, natch) dip and serve it up with gluten-free bagel chips alongside gluten-filled bagel chips, you're going to get glutened. Other people's dipping of the gluten into your dip will wind up in your body. I know! It's the most annoying thing about eating gluten-free. But it's not quite as annoying as pooping out your insides every five minutes. Some more fun examples of cross-contamination include:

• You use the same pasta pot to make your gluten-free pasta right after you made that gluten-filled mac and cheese for the kids.

• You simply scrape that gravy off your mashed potatoes and move on. Not so fast. Unless you're running to the bathroom.

• Someone came over to your house when you were out of town and put his chicken fingers in your oven and on your pan. And now your pan has those stuck-on crunchies attached to its surface like forever. Not that I'm mad or anything, Aaron.

• You pick out the gluten-free Rice Chex from the Chex Mix that includes gluten-filled pretzels and gluten-filled soy sauce.

• Same mixing spoon used for two very different recipes. Obviously one has gluten in it. You get where I'm going here, right?

• You make out with someone who just ate a piece of chocolate cake. (Although honestly, why would you kiss someone who is flaunting his cake-eating abilities in front of you? Plus—get a room.)

All of these examples, as well as those that are clearly labeled on your dip, are ways to get sick even when you think you're eating gluten-free. These reasons are also why some people will tell you to get rid of all of your pots and pans and start over with gluten-free cookware. These same people will suggest you march into everyone's kitchen and demand to see how the food is prepared. Although I appreciate this rigid approach to your health, and it's totally true that it will save your stomach from many woes, I will tell you that I do none of those things.

I do have one pot and strainer that is dedicated to anything gluten-related, and I try to keep the other ones (which were used to cook up big ol' pots of gluten before my diagnosis) clean and gluten-free at all times. I also tossed my wooden spoons and wooden cutting boards because those wooden tools like to hoard gluten. Yet I've also been known to indulge in a bean dip that was made in the same factory as gluten. Many times. Come on, it's yummy, yummy bean dip! Did I get sick? No. Could something have happened inside me that I was not aware of? Of course. In fact, it most surely has. Which is why I will now make the announcement that I'm a risk-taker, a rebel. It's certainly easier for me to find a restaurant to meet up with friends when I have this laissez-faire attitude about cross-contamination. And it's definitely helpful in that I didn't throw out all of my wedding gifts and restock my kitchen once I was diagnosed. But you know what happened to me at my follow-up visit? Flat villi. You don't want that, so listen up.

You've got to make your own choices on how stringent you're going to be regarding cross-contamination, and every doctor will tell you to be ever vigilant. But remember, unless you're in your own kitchen, you can't control everything. Even gluten-free menus are at the mercy of the person preparing your food. Just by going to someone else's kitchen you're taking a chance. Either you're willing to do that, or you are not. Hey, it's cool either way. I understand that my lack of willingness to be a crazed harpy when I walk into a restaurant could cost me a centimeter or two of villi. It's a chance I take, but not one I recommend for everyone. Or hell, anyone. Hence, my "buyer beware" warning. But if you're serious about keeping gluten out of your gut, you've really got to be intense about this. And sometimes, intense means totally annoying. (See Chapter 4.) But hey, who are we kidding? Gluten-free people are already annoying by simply existing. At least according to assholes everywhere.

So Where Do I Find the Doughnuts?

I'm so sorry, but you can't have real doughnuts anymore. Correction: You can have doughnuts that actually taste like cake. Those fluffy, crispy-skinned doughnuts are really not in your future. But I do have a rad recipe for beignets! Although not as poufy as a Krispy Kreme, they do have some air up in them. And they're French! But never fear, in addition to the amazoids recipes found here, there are a ton of gluten-free desserts out there for you to grab and go when you're at the store. You can still have super-delicious desserts that will add just as many (or more!) pounds onto your ass as those with delicious gluten. It's a win/win. Here are a few of my favorite things:

- Ice cream, gelato, sorbet—So long as there aren't any cookie pieces or other add-ins that are covered in gluten, enjoy!

- Flan—Naturally gluten-free, naturally fat-adding. YUM.

- M&Ms—You may find yourself living on these wonders because you can find them anywhere.

- Chocolate-covered almonds—Or any nut, really. Yes, I'm going to say it. Go nuts!

- French macarons—Most of them, anyway. Occasionally some will have gluten, so always ask. (You may be thinking: *Macarons, really? Where, pray tell, do I find macarons in my small province?* Macarons are the hot new "it" dessert, replacing your local cupcake joint as I type. They'll be there, and they will be delicious.)

• Meringues—Fluffy balls of sugar with no gluten. What's not to like?

• Pudding—Not all pudding is created equal, but most brands and flavors are totally gluten-free. That goes for mousse too, which is just fancy pudding.

• Jell-O—Try the many flavors of pudding's cousin from the wrong side of the tracks, Jell-O. You can even enjoy them as a shot! (See the recipes.)

A Short Conversation About Flour

While we're on the topic of making delicious sweets, let's have a frank discussion about gluten-free flour, the basis of most great sweet things. Unlike the dark ages of every day before about four years ago, there are five million gluten-free flour options available to you. It's confusing. You can, and should, experiment with all of these grain flours that are gluten-free, like sorghum, brown rice, tapioca, quinoa, potato, millet, and the new kid on the block, green banana. (Although I'm not experimenting with green banana flour because that is just *weird*.) The idea behind mixing it up with different grain flours is you'll get a nutritional powerhouse by eating healthy grain flours rather than grabbing your basic gluten-free all-purpose flour that usually contains rice flour, cornstarch, potato starch, and maybe xanthan gum. This is a great idea. But let me tell you how this is going to go down. You'll buy all of these exotic flours, experiment once or twice, and abandon them in the back of your cabinet where they'll grow stale or be invaded by weevils and freak you out for life. That's just unhygienic, and quite frankly I don't even know if bugs are gluten-free. OK, bugs *are* totally gluten-free. Still, skip that step and grab the all-purpose. Let's talk about those!

Cup4Cup by Thomas Keller—I made the most amazing Christmas cookies using Cup4Cup Flour, and that's one reason I worship at the altar of Thomas Keller. When you use Cup4Cup gluten-free flour you also don't have to add xanthan gum. So when you look at my recipes, omit the xanthan gum if you're in possession of this fancy flour. However, there's no need to go all fancy-pants when you're battering your mozzarella sticks. Save this white gold for when it really matters, and you're feeling wealthy.

King Arthur's Gluten-Free Multi-Purpose Flour—There's a reason King Arthur's gluten-free multi-purpose flour has a recipe for popovers on the box. Because King Arthur's G-F M-P flour can be used to make some effing delicious popovers. This is a fantastic go-to for just about everything else as well. I've actually (knock on wood) never had anything turn out badly when using King Arthur's multi-purpose gluten-free flour. You do have to add xanthan gum if you're using Art's mix, but you'll always have a stash of that in your cabinets anyway now that you're a mutant.

Bob's Red Mill All-Purpose Gluten-Free Baking Flour—Bob is adorable and from Portland, Oregon. Do you need another reason? OK, here's one: BRM is committed to high-quality and safe products. They rock. Also, they make that xanthan gum I was talking about.

Better Batter Seasoned Flour Mix—If you're frying, this is the way to go. It's like Better Batter knows that what we really want, as gluten-haters, is that thick crunchy coating on our chicken/deep-fried Kool-Aid/broccoli. They are truly mind readers for the gluten-free. Better Batter's cup-for-cup all-purpose flour is also the bomb when you're baking, and you can skip that xanthan gum too.

Some people don't like using the exact cup-for-cup substitutions that are offered by Better Batter and Cup4Cup, but I've had consistent—and delicious—results using these mixtures. In fact, for the most part when I whip up something using either of these direct substitution flours, it's even better than using a mixture of other grain flours plus xanthan gum.

I'm thinking it's time I explained what xanthan gum is all about and why it keeps butting into every conversation. The thing about gluten is that it's incredibly sticky. Once you remove gluten from your baking equation, you've got a lack of sticky situation on your hands. Xanthan gum is a thickening agent in many foodstuffs, from salad dressings to sauces, and it also acts as the sticky when you're using gluten-free flours. Say you have a thing against the letter X; there's also guar gum. Both of these gums are gluten-free and used for the sole purpose of making food stable. Arrowroot is another thickening and sticky agent some chefs add to gluten-free single-grain flours, but it is incredibly expensive. Xanthan gum doesn't have a taste, but wow, does it feel funny. Thank goodness it doesn't feel funny in your mouth because then we'd never eat it and we'd be walking around without gluten-free cake. Xanthan gum gets weird once it comes into contact with liquid; it starts to feel like you're putting on a pair of silky gloves when you wash your hands after handling. But this is the least of your worries when it comes to the unpleasantness of gluten intolerance.

As you read this, there are a zillion other people developing gluten-free all-purpose flours. Experiment and find out how you get the best results in the easiest way possible. Although I'm all for trying every different combination of gluten-free goodness in order to find muffin nirvana, some night you're really just going to need to throw something in flour and deep-fry that sucker within an inch of its gluten-free life. It shouldn't be tougher than your high school chemistry class to make deep-fried goodness. I recommend making life easier and going all-purpose.

Sneaky A-Hole Foods That Have Gluten Even Though You'd Never Know It by Looking

Here's some more bad news, my friends. Gluten is a sneaky bastard. Sometimes you're all "Wow, this gluten-free meal is delicious—oh, damn." It happens to the best of us, and you live and you learn. Just so you don't have as many living-and-learning accidents in your pants as I did, I'm going to fill you in on those not-obvious glutenous foods that are no longer allowed in your gut.

Soy sauce—I don't get this, and I never will. But the sneakiest of all is the soy sauce. Because you don't exactly get that wheat feel when you're dining on sushi. Luckily there is a wheat-free tamari you can buy and carry with you when you head out for rolls. Of course, you have to ask if the plate of raw fish you're about to enjoy already has soy sauce dripping from its shiny loins. For some of you, this is an easy one. You're thinking, "I hate sushi!" Well, my picky friends, soy sauce is also found in marinades, salad dressings, and teriyaki sauce, making it the sneakiest gluten of all. What this means for you is that when you're over at a friend's house or at a restaurant, you have to explain the whole soy sauce thing. Then people will be like, "Wait, can you have tofu?" Because soy sauce sounds exactly like "soy," and people will be confused. Yes, you can have soy products of any kind, so long as they are not dripping in soy sauce. Annoying, I know.

WTF, Triticale?

We're all clear on what wheat, rye, and barley are when we gulp them down. If you're like me, when you heard that gluten intolerants cannot eat triticale you thought, *What in the hell is triticale? A club drug?* Worse. Triticale is the unholy marriage of rye and wheat. Why people felt the need to merge these two grains is beyond me, but I'm sure someone had a good reason. And that good reason was surely cash money. Regardless, here's where you can find triticale, and so here is what you must avoid. Also, look for triticale on cereal labels—especially cereals not made in the United States, because apparently triticale is more of an international crop and not found as frequently in the U.S.A. And so long as no one starts trading their Levi's for triticale seed, we Americans should be OK if we keep our eyes peeled.

- Cereal—Kashi Seven Whole Grain Blend, Bob's Red Mill Triticale Hot Cereal, and more
- Bob's Red Mill—Triticale Flour & Triticale Berries
- *Star Trek*'s "The Trouble with Tribbles"—Seriously, they talked about triticale in that episode. I'm pretty sure you can't get glutened from watching *Star Trek*, but we never can be too careful, can we?

Oats—Oatmeal seemed like an excellent breakfast alternative to me when I was diagnosed with the celiac. No more Cap'n Crunch meant it was time for me to grow up. However, oats can bug a celiac like nobody's business. This is for a few reasons. One, some facilities cut their oats with flour. *Phhhhhpt.* Two, some gluten-intolerant folks find oats to be irritating as well.

Just to be safe, you should buy "pure, uncontaminated oats," and the package must be marked. Even then, only moderate amounts (½ cup to ¾ cup of such oats) are advised. I highly recommend you go out and get these pure oats; otherwise, you'll never be able to make my delicious gluten-free double chocolate oatmeal cookies. (See recipes.)

Soups—How did that yummy soup get so thick? Gluten. You know what else gets glutened to make them thick? Marinades, gravies, salad dressings, and sauces. Yes, even the next one.

Enchilada sauce—Yeah, I didn't even think this was a thing. It's a sauce, made from peppers and tomatoes. However, as I discovered, some enchilada sauce also has chicken broth, so vegetarians are not safe either. Let this be the lesson to all sensitive types: Any food that has a barcode must be considered suspect.

Play-Doh—If you were like me, you totally ate Play-Doh as a kid. Oh, you didn't? Well, don't start now because it has gluten in it.

Beer—Maybe beer is not so sneaky because it seemed to me that everyone warned me off having a cold one when I was first diagnosed. (Was it something I did?) But you may not automatically think of beer as having gluten. It does. Don't drink it. Unless it's gluten-free beer, but some of those even sneak some gluten inside, so read that label and/or call that beer company.

Communion Wafers—Sorry, religious folks who partake in the body of Christ, but you're going to be benched. Ask your priest or minister about providing an alternative or risk the wrath of the Lord.

Dextrin—What is this, you may ask? It's a sneaky starch that's used as a thickener and in medications. Yep, it's got gluten.

Baking Powder—Seriously, how annoying is that? Look for the gluten-free label on that staple.

Skinny Vanilla Lattes—Yep, learned that the hard way. Asshole mermaid.

Stamps and Envelopes—Hahahahahahaha. As if you use those anymore.

Vitamins and Medication—This one is a doozy. You need vitamins to make sure your new gluten-free self is getting all of the nutrients your sensitive body requires. Yet some vitamins and medications have gluten. Dang it! As for any medication you're taking, don't risk just reading the ingredients list, also ask the pharmacist. If s/he seems clueless, call the manufacturer.

Seriously, you don't want to give up normal good-tasting pizza just to get glutened by your cold medicine. Don't rely on a generic of a trusted medication either. I found myself getting glutened repeatedly by my generic Tylenol because the brand name is gluten-free. Turns out some of those generics (Safeway brand, I'm looking at you) throw some wheat starch in there without telling us, or rather, without a warning label. Never assume; you know what they say about that.

Malt—Whether it's that delicious one from the *shoppe* or the weird one at Long John Silver's, anything with the word "malt" is now forbidden because malt usually means barley malt.

Mustard—Not all mustard, but some types are made with ale. That's beer, if you're an American. Again, you've gotta read that label and/or call the company. I know! Your phone bill is getting ridiculous.

Licorice—And just as I moved to the land of Red Vines. This also goes for licorice flavoring.

Lunch Meat—Some brands of cold cuts, like Boar's Head, pride themselves on being gluten-free. Others are chock full of fillers. Fillers with gluten. Is your phone ready for more action? Call 'em.

Touching Bagels—OK, most of you know that you can't eat bagels anymore. Obvious gluten source, am I right? I discovered the hard way ("the hard way" means pooping like crazy with a house full of guests I had just fed breakfast) that even touching a bagel can trigger an attack. I don't know if it's because bagels are jam-packed with gluten ~~or I licked my hands after~~ or have a secret weapon that shoots bagelness into your bloodstream just by standing near, but we can no longer have bagels in our house that could possibly come into contact with any part of my body. That's right, *any* part. (Note: Since you have to actually ingest gluten to get sick, I certainly touched a bagel and licked my hand because I'm disgusting like that. So just don't touch a bagel, in case of the licking. If you must touch a bagel, wash your hands and lick away.)

Your takeaway here is this: Anything that comes with a label or in a package must be treated as suspect. If it is not food in its purest form (and its purest form is not wheat, rye, barley, or triticale), you've got to figure out exactly what was used in the making of said food. Everyone has been lying to us about salad being good for us because salad has so many places to hide the gluten. Gluten is a fiend and must be ferreted out. Now you know why some people only eat steak and broccoli.

Do I Have Cancer?
And Other Joys of Being a Celiac

If you're diagnosed with celiac, you may have other things to worry about if you don't banish gluten from your presence. How much do we really need to worry, on a scale of "Starting a bucket list RIGHT NOW" to "Really? So I have a better chance of marrying a terrorist?" Well, if you cut gluten out of your diet you can dramatically decrease the chances of your developing one of these horrible diseases that are complications resulting from untreated celiac. In fact, the best way to keep these diseases far away from your body is to go gluten-free and stay that way. Then you've got a better chance of being killed in a car accident. This is the feel-good part of the book, obviously. Ready to be scared straight?

- Malnutrition
- Anemia
- Osteoporosis
- Rickets
- Lymphoma
- Bowel cancer
- Peripheral neuropathy
- Seizures
- Thyroid disease

More Lies About Gluten

Here's another thing about sneaky gluten: People also love to lie about it. Sometimes that lie comes in the form of "There isn't any gluten in this fried wonton, I swear," and other times it comes in the form of the alarmist who declares there is gluten in every single thing you eat except for that magical quinoa. I'm sorry to tell you this, my gluten-free friends, but there are people on the Internet who lie. Hence, my total freakout about ChapStick when I was convinced that lovely lip balm was the cause of all of my problems because someone on the Internet swore ChapStick contained gluten. FYI, it doesn't, so keep those lips moisturized without fear. The same thing happened when someone else on the Internet (or maybe it's the same horrible person) announced that you could only drink potato vodka and that otherwise vodka has gluten. Seriously, these people want to take away your ChapStick and vodka on top of all of the other deliciousness. These are evil people. Instead of talking to the Internet, talk to a nutritionist. Which is what I did, and now my lips are totally smooth again, and I'm drunk.

Shazi Shabatian is an amazing registered dietitian who first introduced me to the concept of "crazy things that may have gluten inside" when I met with her after my diagnosis. She was nice enough to give me the straight dope. Although Shabatian has been doing this dietitian business for twenty years, she is adamant that "the science remains the same" even though the product market for gluten-free goods has exploded. "The foods we were to stay away from then are the foods we are to stay away from now," she explains. "So what really gets my goat is gluten misinformation. People get confused and really restrict their diet and are at even greater risk for nutritional imbalances. Please learn the facts (like vodka is distilled, which removes gluten), so next time you read something somewhere, you are able to distinguish between truth and hype."

The danger, as Shabatian just explained, is that if you start taking more things out of your diet you could wind up being even unhealthier than you were before you started cleaning out your cupboards. We need a variety of foods in our lives, but sadly gluten will not be one of them. Keep on knocking other stuff out of the park and it's just going to be you and your sad head of broccoli left at the table. You heard it here, folks: Go drink vodka. And all of you Internet hoaxers need to go back to trolling the Huffington Post.

But who am I kidding? It's an Internet world, and we all immediately go to Dr. Google the second we have a question about our health. I do it too, but after digging in to real research that doesn't start with an http, I've realized that you can't allow your health to depend on charlie3676. The best way to get your gluten questions answered is to a) Read this book (duh); b) Ignore anyone who swears there is gluten in something and follows that proclamation by one or more exclamation points; and c) Call your dietitian. You don't want to have your birthday night ruined because some know-it-all swears that wine contains gluten because she read it on www.imaglutenliar.com. Who invited that jerk, anyway?

So What Kind of Weird Stores Sell Gluten-Free Stuff?

If you guessed Whole Foods, you're totally a winner! Except for that whole bank account thing because you will soon be the biggest loser in that arena. But I'm not going to knock Whole Foods because that is one of the only places I know I can go and get food for the norms (aka my family) and food for me. It's a beautiful place, even if we had to give up two years of family vacation in order for me to shop there.

Other great stores that stock up on the gluten-free include:

- Erewhon
- Gelson's
- H-E-B/Central Market
- Stop & Shop
- Trader Joe's
- Vons/Safeway

- Wegmans

- Wheatsville

- Wild Oats

If you have a local food co-op now might be the time to join. I say "might be" because you do have lots of other options, but food co-ops are traditionally the keepers of the alternative foods. The keepers of bizarre politics (on all sides—not knocking anyone's POV in particular) and member infighting too, unless you're super lucky to be involved in one of those food co-ops that allows you to pay extra to not deal. I've also heard rumors about totally lovely food co-op situations. I've just never seen them in real life. And never, ever, ever forget to shop at your local farmers' market. Just skip the deep-fried homemade pita chips. Dammit.

Luckily there are also exclusive gluten-free markets also popping up around the country. My local favorite is Pam MacD's in Burbank. Do you know what it feels like to walk into a grocery store and know that you can eat every single thing in that sucker? It feels good. Real good.

If you're not so lucky, and your local Albertsons has not gotten with the program either (because many of the big chains are also on this expensive-food gravy train), there's always the online shop. Even Amazon can help you stock up on gluten-free food, but there are online specialty stores as well. (See Resources.)

Now that you've identified your local purveyor of gluten-free food, congratulations! You are totally a member of the food awareness cult. Maybe you thought these people were annoying before, but guess what? *You're totally one of them now.*

Don't Forget Your Vitamins

Now you know what to cut out of your diet, and like any major change in what you consume, your nutritional balance is about to be way off. If you have celiac, your villi may be so damaged that you're not absorbing vitamins from your food at all, which means you've got two problems. It's a long road back to health for those crazy villi, so you'll also need to get your multivitamin in while your gut is healing. Your doctor should be running blood tests on you to see where you may be deficient—vitamin-wise—and those are the vitamins and/or minerals you've got to put back into your body as well, so you can be healthy again. At the same time consider what nutrients you will be losing when you are no longer eating gluten. This reconnaissance work is especially important to undertake for children who are no longer consuming bread that has been fortified with vitamins and minerals and are still growing.

My nutritionist recommended I take not only a multivitamin but a calcium and magnesium supplement as well. Silly me, I thought maybe I could take these vitamins for a few months and then I'd be all set. Since I have celiac, I'll most likely never be "all set," so my personal vitamin train keeps running. Everyone is different in his or her nutritional needs, so don't leave your doctor's office without knowing what is exactly right for your body as well. Don't forget to get a brand recommendation because, as you've seen in the sneaky gluten section, many vitamins also contain gluten. The last thing you need while trying to heal is to sabotage your body with vitamin gluten.

In a perfect world, you'll simply add the right foods to your diet to replace what your body has been missing. We live in a very imperfect world filled with meetings, travel, stress, and time constraints. I personally live in an imperfect world filled with delicious gluten-free muffins that are much more appealing than quinoa. Supplementing with vitamins is now crucial for your well-being. Certainly vitamins cannot replace whole foods that give you the proper nutrients, but they can help your body feel OK once more and help to defend your body against illness.

Chapter Three

RECIPES FOR THE
Downtrodden
(AKA THE GLUTEN-FREE)

Now that you understand that gluten must get out of your life, you're about to go through major withdrawal. You need to stuff those bad feelings with cheese, fried gluten-free goodness, and sugar. That is, if you're like me. If you're not like me, you might want to flip to Chapter 5, where you can learn how to be vegan and gluten-free. But back to me.

There are some really fantastic gluten-free cookbooks out there. I know this because I bought them and then decided to heck with it, I was not going to mix and match twenty-eight gluten-free flour blends while I was experimenting with pie. You might want to do this eventually, but in the beginning you really need some easy gluten-free recipes that won't make you sweat. Which is why you should grab one of those all-purpose gluten-free flours I was going on about and several sticks of butter.

This is where I warn you that you could put on some serious weight as you experiment with the gluten-free diet. Maybe that's a good thing, given your recent dramatic weight loss. Maybe that's a bad thing, and at some point you'll look southward and wonder if you accidentally ingested a puppy. But that's OK because right now you're dealing with deprivation and the pain of becoming that person no one wants to dine out with anymore. You need the comfort only a gluten-free cupcake can give you. And someday, when you're ready, you'll realize that you're all over that dark period and you can enjoy a gluten-free gluttony moment every now and then instead of every five minutes. Apparently that's progress.

When I realized I had to go gluten-free, my southern and Cajun roots damn near shriveled up and died. I made it my mission to re-create family recipes in the gluten-free style, dammit. And luckily, my mother had put together a makeshift family cookbook back when printing your own books was just coming into style. I have my very own copy of *Recipes from Our Family Tree* with this inscription on the inside cover:

Christmas 1992

April,

I know cooking is not one of your favorite things to do, but I think you'll find some foods in here you can make as well as eat. (Look in the cookie section) In case you find new recipes to add to the family collection, there's plenty of room on the back of the pages.

Love,
Mom

In response to the taunting about the cookies, I'd like to point out that my cookbook is being published without a plastic ring holding the pages together. Boo-ya, family! I'm cooking! Although that particular cookbook did have a few recipes "by April"—yes, Rice Krispie treats count—most of these gems are old-school and with a southern bent. For me, that's total comfort food, and if the glut of restaurants opening up everywhere serving mac and cheese is any indication, it's pretty dang comforting for everyone. Now, I've made it all gluten-free. Go crazy, my people.

Before we hit the kitchen, let's talk about the changes you'll discover when you remove the gluten from your kitchen. I don't want to shock you, but life will never be the same again. Oh no, you're totally in shock now, right? Read these tips and take control over your out-of-control situation.

Gluten-Free Cooking Tips

• Some sad news about gluten-free cake and cookie batter: It sucks. You don't want to eat it, or the acrid taste will stick to the roof of your mouth and you will not be able to enjoy that lovely Italian cream cake you just made. Don't be tempted. And I'm sorry. But hey, at least your risk of salmonella decreases.

• A word about frying. There are people in this world who own deep-fat fryers, and there are people who do not. I am in the former category, and that's how I like to fry up my food. I've included instructions for pan-frying because I totally get that some of you are not evolved enough to own your own personal fry basket. It's cool. But if you own a deep fryer, you can see how frying food at a high temperature for a smaller amount of time is a guaranteed crisper-upper and is totally delicious. Just sayin'.

• You know when recipes start out with preheat? It's even more important for the gluten-free baking, which is why I always put it first. Preheat your oven for at least twenty minutes so you will always have a hot oven. It already takes gluten-free baked goods longer to cook, but to get the right combo of cooked through without burning the edges, you really need to start hot.

• Don't be afraid to experiment with liquid. I find that some gluten-free flours are a bit drier than others and require more liquid. I also find that some pancake mixes and cake mixes become too liquefied if I add the amount of milk, water, or oil on the instructions. Don't be afraid to tinker if you feel like something is not right.

• If you are using a cup-for-cup type gluten-free flour (Cup4Cup, Better Batter) for baking, omit the xanthan gum, since it is included in those mixes. Additionally, I've found that if I'm baking something more delicate like crêpes or cookies, using these cup-for-cup flours gives me a better result.

• There's a reason you find gluten-free baked goods in the freezer section of your store. Gluten-free baked goods do not keep for long periods of time. Or rather, they dry out a lot quicker than traditional gluten-filled goodies. So eat fast, or freeze.

Let's eat!

Breakfast

. . . .

Lemon Ricotta Pancakes

One of the first food items I panicked about was the almighty pancake. Since I had perfected this recipe before I went all g-free, I immediately experimented to see if it could be as awesome using straight-up gluten-free all-purpose flour. Guess what? IT STILL ROCKS.

Prep time: 10 minutes **Cook time:** 7 minutes
Makes: 8 pancakes

INGREDIENTS

1½ cups all-purpose gluten-free flour
1 teaspoon xanthan gum
2 tablespoons sugar
1 teaspoon baking soda
½ teaspoon salt
1½ cups buttermilk
2 large eggs, separated
1 tablespoon grated lemon zest
⅓ cup ricotta
Vegetable oil
Butter, for serving (optional)
Syrup, for serving (optional)

1. In a large bowl, sift together the gluten-free flour, xanthan gum, sugar, baking soda, and salt.

2. In a medium bowl, whisk the buttermilk, egg yolks, and lemon zest to combine.

3. Stir the buttermilk mixture into the flour mixture until just evenly moistened. Gently stir in the ricotta until thoroughly combined.

4. In the bowl of a stand mixer fitted with the whisk attachment, beat the egg whites on high speed until soft peaks form. Gently fold the egg whites into the batter until just incorporated.

5. Heat the vegetable oil over medium-high heat on a griddle or frying pan. When hot, turn the heat down to medium and drop ½-cup portions of batter onto the griddle or pan. Cook until bubbles start to appear on surface of the pancake—about 2 to 3 minutes—then turn the pancakes with a wide spatula and brown the other side, cooking 2 to 3 minutes longer. Coat pan with more oil as necessary to cook remaining pancakes.

6. Serve with butter and syrup or plain.

Aunt Loretta's Breakfast Casserole

One of Aunt Loretta's skills is always being prepared when overnight guests arrive unexpectedly. From her kitchen comes a delicious breakfast casserole that I have since turned gluten-free. Loretta might be appalled that we eat this on any occasion, as one should be when you see the amount of sausage in this recipe, but it's so good my family cannot resist pretending we have overnight guests biweekly.

Luckily, it's one of those recipes in which the gluten-free bread soaks up so much of the rest of the casserole, you can't tell the difference. This means you don't need to make your own bread for this recipe, just pick up a loaf at your local gluten-free friendly shop.

Prep time: 20 minutes + overnight **Cook time:** 45 minutes
Makes: 10 servings

INGREDIENTS

1 pound gluten-free sausage (check with your butcher, or on the
   package, that it is gluten-free)
6 eggs
2 cups milk
1 teaspoon salt
1 teaspoon dry mustard
6 slices of gluten-free bread, broken into chunks
1½ cups shredded sharp cheddar

Note: Prepare this casserole the night before you plan to serve it.

1. Brown the gluten-free sausage. Transfer it to a paper towel–lined bowl to drain off excess fat and let the sausage cool.

2. In a large bowl, beat the eggs and milk together. Add the salt and mustard and beat well to combine. Add the bread and stir until it softens. Stir in shredded cheese and cooled sausage.

3. Pour the batter into a greased 9-by-13-inch baking dish. Cover with plastic wrap and refrigerate overnight.

4. The next day, preheat the oven to 350°F. Remove the baking dish from the refrigerator, and bake the casserole for 40 to 45 minutes. Serve warm.

. . . .

Beignets

Since my diagnosis, I've avoided going back to New Orleans. Why? Those damned delicious beignets. Once you've gone Café Du Monde, you're never the same. In fact, I used to hunt down Café Du Monde beignet mix when I lived in New York City and made the beignets in my deep fryer, but I never thought I would be able to enjoy the sugar-sprinkled taste of a French dough-nut ever again. I was wrong.

It was pretty much the most amazing day ever when I introduced gluten-free beignets to my household. Just a few comments from the family who acted as my taste-testers: "This is the best beignet ever!" "I love beignets!" "Your recipe made beignets better!" And my favorite, "Doughnuts can be circle AND square."

Prep time: 2½ hours **Cook time:** 10 minutes
Makes: 35 beignets

INGREDIENTS

1½ cups lukewarm water
½ cup sugar
1¼ teaspoons salt
¼ ounce active dry yeast
2 eggs
1 cup evaporated milk
3 cups all-purpose gluten-free flour
4 cups gluten-free pancake mix
¼ cup vegetable shortening
2 (32-ounce) bottles of vegetable oil, to fill the fryer
3 cups confectioners' sugar

1. Combine the water, sugar, salt, and yeast in a large bowl, and set the mixture aside to sit for 10 minutes.

2. Beat the eggs and evaporated milk together, then stir in the yeast mixture until combined.

3. In a separate bowl, sift the gluten-free flour and pancake mix together. Slowly add the flour mixture to the egg mixture, then thoroughly mix in the vegetable shortening.

4. Place dough on a surface floured with gluten-free flour and knead it until smooth. Place the dough in a large, clean bowl, cover it with a clean dish towel, and allow the dough to rise for at least two hours.

5. After the dough has risen, place it on the floured surface and roll it out to about ¼ inch thick. Cut the dough into 1-inch squares.

6. Fill a deep fryer with vegetable oil or pour enough oil into a deep skillet to cover the entire beignet. Preheat the fryer on the medium-high setting (if using a skillet, heat the oil over medium-high heat). Fry the dough squares in batches, being careful not to crowd the fryer or pan and making sure the beignets fry to a golden brown on all sides.

7. While the beignets cook, place the confectioners' sugar in a bowl.

8. Remove the beignets from the oil and drain them on a paper towel–covered plate to absorb excess oil, then immediately roll them in confectioners' sugar to coat. Serve warm.

. . . .

Prize Coffee Cake with Streusel Filling

We have two different recipes for coffee cake in our family cookbook. One is just plain old coffee cake (sorry, Aunt Margaret), and then there's the "prize-winning" version that Grandmother Reeves would bust out.

This version, with the streusel, is far superior—and easily made gluten-free. Not to get all high and mighty on you (OK, a little), but I also made this when I was in 4-H, and I will tell you that our prize-winning streak at the county fair was multigenerational.

Prep time: 10 minutes **Cook time:** 35 minutes
Makes: 9 servings

INGREDIENTS

For the Streusel:
½ cup brown sugar
2 tablespoons all-purpose gluten-free flour
2 teaspoons cinnamon
2 tablespoons butter, melted
½ cup pecans, chopped

For the Cake:
¾ cup sugar
¼ cup vegetable shortening
1 egg
½ cup milk
1½ cups all-purpose gluten-free flour
¼ teaspoon xanthan gum
2 teaspoons baking powder
½ teaspoon salt

1. Preheat the oven to 375°F.

2. Make the streusel: Combine the brown sugar, gluten-free flour, cinnamon, melted butter, and pecans in a medium bowl. Set aside.

3. Make the cake: Beat the sugar, shortening, and egg together. Add the milk and beat well to combine.

4. Sift the flour, xanthan gum, baking powder, and salt together. Gradually add the flour mixture to the milk mixture and beat well to combine.

5. Pour half the batter into a greased 9-inch square or round pan. Sprinkle half the streusel mixture over the batter. Add the remaining batter, then top with the remaining streusel mixture.

6. Bake for 35 minutes. Serve warm.

Snacks & Apps

. . . .

Sweet Potato Chips with Chive Crème Fraîche

As you know, any snack in a bag can be suspect to the gluten intolerant. Which is why your deep fryer should become your new BFF. I ~~love~~ hate to keep harping on that point, but it's true.

Whether it's sweet potatoes, gluten-free tortillas cut into those cute little triangle shapes, or anything, really, frying simply makes it better. Also, it's super-duper easy to make a crispy, salty snack that won't send you running to the bathroom. Win!

This simple crème fraîche dip can be trotted out at any time as well. Super easy, yet super impressive.

Prep time: 5 minutes   **Cook time:** 8 minutes per batch
Makes: 6 servings

INGREDIENTS

Vegetable oil
2 large sweet potatoes
Salt
Freshly ground black pepper
Paprika
1½ cup crème fraîche
1 tablespoon chopped chives

1. Fill a deep fryer with vegetable oil or pour enough oil into a deep skillet to cover the sweet potato slices. Preheat the fryer on high (if using a skillet, heat the oil over medium-high heat).

2. Leaving the skin on, thinly slice sweet potatoes using a mandoline or a very sharp knife.

3. Place handfuls of potato slices into the oil and fry until crispy, 5 to 8 minutes. If you're using a skillet, turn the potato slices after 3 minutes to fry the opposite side.

4. Remove the chips from the oil, and drain them on a paper towel–covered plate to absorb excess oil. Transfer the chips to a serving basket and sprinkle them with salt, pepper, and paprika to taste.

5. Combine the crème fraîche and chives. Serve the crème fraîche dip alongside the chips.

· ·

Curry Bagel Chips

The rumors about gluten-free bagels and bread are true. You need to toast them within an inch of their lives to get them to that gluteny goodness. Which is why making bagel chips is the perfect thing to do with your gluten-free bagels.

Bake 'em, spice 'em, and serve 'em up with some inventive hummus or a lovely dip. You will not give two craps about what those gluten-eaters are eating over there when you crunch on these flavorful chips.

Prep time: 10 minutes **Cook time:** 25 minutes
Makes: 12 servings

INGREDIENTS

3 gluten-free bagels
⅓ cup olive oil
2 tablespoons mustard seeds

1 tablespoon curry powder
2 tablespoons cumin

1. Preheat the oven to 350°F. Slice the gluten-free bagels from top to bottom into very thin rounds. Set aside.

2. In a small skillet, heat the olive oil over low heat. Add the mustard seeds and listen closely for a pop, which is how you know the mustard seeds have released their sharp, nutty, delicious flavor.

3. Remove the oil from the heat and transfer it to a bowl. Mix in the curry powder and cumin.

4. Place the bagel slices in the bowl with the oil and spices and toss to coat. Transfer the bagel chips to a baking sheet and bake for 20 minutes, or until golden brown and crispy.

. . . .

Super Tex Nachos

Oh, jeez, I love nachos. When you love something so much, you're quite likely to eat it without care, which is never a good idea when you're gluten-free. Which is why I perfected my own mouthwatering nachos at home, where I control every single ingredient.

I don't use refried beans from a can but instead whip up my own. You can use chips you fry yourself without worrying about cross-contamination, and top it all off with fresh guacamole like the pros make. Once you go all fresh, you'll never go back. That is, until you find yourself starving in front of your local On The Border.

Prep time: 15 minutes **Cook time:** 20 minutes
Makes: One big-ass plate of nachos

INGREDIENTS

For the Refried Beans:
1 tablespoon olive oil
1 shallot, diced
1 clove of garlic, diced
2 cups pinto or black beans, cooked from dry or canned
½ jalapeño pepper, deseeded and diced
1 teaspoon cumin
2 teaspoons cayenne pepper
Juice of 1 lime

For the Tortilla Chips:
1 to 2 cups vegetable oil for frying
6 to 8 gluten-free corn tortillas
Sea salt

For the Guacamole:
1 ripe avocado
½ red onion, diced
1 clove of garlic, or 2 teaspoons garlic powder
1 tablespoon cumin
2 teaspoons diced jalapeño pepper
1 to 2 teaspoons cayenne pepper, to taste
2 tablespoons lemon juice
Salt
Freshly ground black pepper
¾ cup grated sharp cheddar
2 tablespoons salsa

1. Make the refried beans: In a medium saucepan over medium heat, heat the olive oil. Add the shallot and garlic and cook until soft and slightly brown.

2. Stir the beans into the sautéed shallots and garlic. Add the jalapeño, cumin, cayenne, and lime juice, and cook over medium heat for about 5 minutes. When beans are well mixed and well cooked, use a potato masher to mash the mixture. Turn the heat to low and let the refried beans simmer while you make the tortilla chips and guacamole.

3. Make the tortilla chips: Heat the vegetable oil in a deep skillet over medium-high heat. The oil should be able to fully cover the chips; you may need to replenish while cooking. (Alternatively, bust out that deep fryer.)

4. Cut each tortilla into fours and place one piece in the oil so you know when the oil is hot enough. Add the tortilla quarters to the oil in batches, being careful not to crowd the pan, and cook until brown. Flip the tortilla quarters with a slotted spoon, then remove them from the oil and drain them on a paper towel–lined plate to absorb excess oil. Sprinkle the tortilla chips with sea salt while they are still warm, then transfer to a large plate to cool. Repeat with the remaining tortilla quarters.

5. Make the guacamole: Cut the avocado in half and remove the pit. Peel away the avocado skin, then slice the flesh in pieces. Place the flesh in a medium bowl and add the onion, garlic, cumin, jalapeño, and cayenne. Add the lemon juice and salt and pepper to taste.

6. Assemble the nachos: Stack the chips, beans, cheese, and a drizzle of salsa, to taste, on a plate or serving platter. Top with the guacamole, and dig right in.

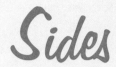

Sides

Crispy Garlic Smashed Potatoes

Another recipe from an amazing restaurant that I totally can't go to now that I can't eat gluten. Umami Burger is a chain known for its secret ingredients. As we all know, secret ingredients = likely gluten poisoning.

I gazed upon the wonder of the smashed potatoes at Umami Burger then later went home and smashed some up my own dang self. It's no secret that these crispy potatoes are delicious.

Prep time: 5 minutes **Cook time:** 45 minutes
Makes: 4 servings

INGREDIENTS

15 new potatoes
2 tablespoons olive oil
Salt
Freshly ground black pepper
2 teaspoons black truffle oil
Parsley or chives, chopped (optional)
Sour cream (optional)

1. Preheat the oven to 450°F.

2. Bring a large pot of water to boil with a pinch of salt. Make sure there is enough water to cover the potatoes. Add the potatoes and boil them until you can pierce them with a fork with little resistance, 15 to 20 minutes.

3. Drain the potatoes and place them, evenly spaced, on a foil-covered baking sheet. Allow to cool for a few minutes, then take a clean dish towel and press on each potato to smash it, but still keep the potato intact.

4. Drizzle olive oil evenly over the smashed potatoes. Season with salt, pepper, and a small amount of black truffle oil. Top with some chopped parsley, chives, or another herb of your choice, if you like. Bake for 25 to 30 minutes, or until crispy.

5. Use a spatula to remove each potato. Serve with sour cream, if desired.

. . . .

Mexican Corn Bread

Why would you take something that is already perfect and mess with it? Because this is my mama's Mexican corn bread, that's why. This cheesy, peppery, moist corn bread rules and will impress your guests.

Also, you can't trust restaurant or store-made corn bread to be gluten-free, so you're now on your own. Try this delicious version with chili or chicken, or for breakfast, or whatever makes you happy.

Prep time: 7 minutes **Cook time:** 45 minutes
Makes: 8 servings

INGREDIENTS

1½ cups gluten-free cornmeal
3 teaspoons baking powder
1 teaspoon salt
2 eggs, beaten
2/3 cup vegetable oil
1 cup buttermilk
3 jalapeños, seeded and chopped
2 cups creamed corn
1 cup grated sharp cheddar

1. Preheat the oven to 350°F.

2. In a large bowl, combine all ingredients except the cheddar. Do not over-mix the batter.

3. Pour half the batter into a greased 9-inch square baking pan. Cover with half the cheddar, then pour in remaining batter and top with the remaining cheese. Bake for 45 minutes.

. . . .

Country Fried Corn with Bacon

This is one of those Oklahoma recipes that have yet to sweep the nation, for reasons way beyond my comprehension. You can't help but get completely addicted to this bacon-fried corn. I would say this bacon corn is like crack, but I don't come from Baltimore. So I'll say like meth.

Prep time: 15 minutes **Cook time:** 25 minutes
Makes: 10 servings

INGREDIENTS

6 ears of corn
8 strips of bacon
2 teaspoons sugar
1 teaspoon salt
1/8 teaspoon freshly ground black pepper
1/2 cup half-and-half

1. Bring 8 quarts of water to a rolling boil in a large stockpot. Place the corn in the rapidly boiling water for 3 minutes, then remove and allow to cool. Remove the corn kernels from the cob with a sharp knife and set aside.

2. Fry the bacon in a large skillet over medium-high heat. Remove the bacon

from the skillet and place on a paper towel–lined plate to drain excess oil and cool the bacon. Reserve 2 tablespoons of the bacon drippings in the skillet.

3. With the skillet over low heat, add the corn, sugar, salt, and pepper to the bacon drippings. Cover, increase the heat to medium, and fry on medium heat for 5 minutes, stirring occasionally.

4. Add the half-and-half and turn the heat to medium-low. Simmer, covered, for 8 to 10 minutes, until the milk is absorbed. Serve hot.

· ·

Baked Cheese & Chive Grits

An incredibly easy Southern dish. My mother used to make these baked cheese grits as a delicious starchy side. I've added chives because I'm fancy like that, and I have tons of chives growing in my herb garden. The chives add a little extra flavor and foodie snootiness to your table. Which is, of course, awesome.

Bob's Red Mill has fantastic gluten-free grits, and you can also use polenta (which I'm pretty sure is Italian for "grits").

Prep time: 5 minutes **Cook time:** 30 minutes
Makes: 10 servings

INGREDIENTS

1 tablespoon salt
2 cups gluten-free grits
1 tablespoon freshly ground black pepper
2 teaspoons sea salt
2 cups grated cheddar
2 tablespoons chopped chives

1. Preheat the oven to 350°F. Bring 6 cups of water to a boil with the salt.

2. Gradually add the gluten-free grits to the boiling water, stirring constantly. Bring the grits to a simmer and stir regularly. Cook until the grits have thickened, about 20 minutes.

3. Transfer the grits to a 2-quart baking dish. Mix in the pepper, sea salt, cheddar, and chives.

4. Bake for 10 minutes.

. . . .

Sweet Kugel

Hands down, one of the best things about Hanukkah is the kugel. Or as I call it in my multicultural home, "mac and cheese with sugar." This is the sweet kugel recipe I've been making since before I had to make it celiac friendly. The only change is shelling out for the gluten-free noodles, and—sorry, if you love raisins—removing the raisins. OK, that has nothing to do with going gluten-free and everything to do with the fact that I hate raisins. Throw some in before your last mix if you have to have those wrinkled grapes.

Prep time: 15 minutes **Cook time:** 1 hour
Makes: 15 servings

INGREDIENTS

16 ounces cottage cheese
16 ounces sour cream
1 cup sugar
5 eggs, beaten
½ cup butter, melted
1 tablespoon vanilla extract
1 (8- to 12-ounce) package gluten-free noodles, cooked, rinsed, and drained
1 tablespoon cinnamon sugar

1. Preheat the oven to 350°F. Butter a 13-by-9-inch baking dish.

2. Mix all ingredients except noodles and cinnamon sugar until well blended. Stir in gluten-free noodles.

3. Spoon the mixture into the prepared dish and sprinkle the top with the cinnamon sugar.

4. Bake for 50 to 60 minutes or until the center is set. Let cool for at least 10 minutes before serving.

. . . .

Potato Latkes

Skip the matzo when you're busting out your latkes for eight days of celebration, and make it a miraculous gluten-free holiday this Hanukkah. Or just whip these up any time of year and call them what my mom does: potato pancakes. Either way, super-duper fried goodness for your gluten-free belly.

Prep time: 20 minutes **Cook time:** 10 minutes per batch
Makes: 15 latkes

INGREDIENTS

1 to 2 pounds potatoes
¾ cup finely chopped onion
1 large egg, lightly beaten
1 teaspoon salt
¾ cup olive oil
Applesauce, for serving
Sour cream, for serving

1. Preheat the oven to 250°F.

2. Peel the potatoes and coarsely grate them by hand, transferring the grated potato to a large bowl of cold water as you work. Soak the grated potatoes for 1 to 2 minutes after the last batch is added to the water, then drain well in a colander.

3. Spread the grated potatoes and the onion on a kitchen towel and roll it up tightly. Twist the towel to wring out as much liquid as possible. Transfer the potato mixture to a bowl and stir in the egg and salt.

4. Heat ¼ cup of the oil in a large skillet over medium-high heat until hot but not smoking. Working in batches, spoon 4 tablespoons potato mixture per latke into the skillet, spreading it into rounds with a fork. Reduce the heat to medium and cook until the undersides are browned, about 5 minutes. Turn the latkes over and cook until the other side is browned, about 5 minutes more. Transfer the latkes to paper towels to drain and season them with salt. Repeat with the remaining potato mixture, adding more oil to the skillet as needed. Keep the finished latkes warm in the oven.

5. Serve with applesauce and sour cream.

Main Course

The Most Amazing Mac & Cheese You'll Ever Eat

I've made this down-and-dirty, nonfancy but delicious mac and cheese so many times since my diagnosis that I'm starting to think I should be embarrassed. All right, I'll be honest. I made this mac and cheese on every occasion I could think of before my diagnosis. I just made some gluten-free substitutions afterward because there was no way I was giving up this yellow gold. And I wonder how I gained so much weight. These are Velveeta thighs, obviously.

Prep time: 25 minutes **Cook time:** 30 minutes
Makes: 10 servings

INGREDIENTS

1 pound gluten-free elbow macaroni
4 tablespoons unsalted butter
$1/3$ cup all-purpose gluten-free flour
4 cups milk, heated
2 cups shredded extra-sharp cheddar
2 cups finely chopped American cheese
Salt
Freshly ground black pepper
Hot pepper sauce
$1/4$ cup freshly grated Parmesan

1. Bring a large pot of lightly salted water to boil over high heat. Add the gluten-free elbow macaroni and cook until al dente. Drain well.

2. Position a rack in the center of the oven and preheat the oven to 350°F. Butter a deep 4-quart casserole dish.

3. Melt the 4 tablespoons of butter in a medium saucepan over medium heat. Whisk in the gluten-free flour. Gradually whisk in the milk. Bring to a simmer, stirring constantly, until the sauce thickens. Reduce the heat to low and simmer for 5 minutes.

4. Remove from the heat and stir in 1 cup each of the cheddar and the American cheese. Season to taste with the salt, pepper, and hot sauce.

5. Combine the remaining cheddar and American cheeses. Spread one-third of the pasta over the bottom of the casserole dish. Top with half of the shredded cheese and a third of the sauce. Repeat, using another third of the pasta, the remaining cheese, and half of the remaining sauce. Finish with the remaining pasta and sauce. Sprinkle Parmesan evenly over the top.

6. Bake until bubbly and golden brown around the edges, about 30 minutes.

. . . .

Chicken-Fried Steak & Gravy

One meal I've been able to make since I was in junior high is the holy trinity of chicken-fried steak, mashed potatoes, and gravy. Granted, I don't eat it as often now that I've passed the age of twenty-one and my metabolism no longer allows for such deliciousness on a weekly basis. But this was tops on my list to make gluten-free once I had to go there.

Some parts of the country make it difficult for you to get your cube steak on. Try a skirt steak if you live where people are more likely to grill fajitas than smother their meat in gravy. I feel for you (and me).

For consistent results when I'm frying something savory, I grab Better Batter gluten-free seasoned flour because it always seems to coat really well and give me that thick heart-attack fry I'm looking for. Plus, you don't need to season the batter.

Prep time: 20 minutes **Cook time:** 17 minutes
Makes: 4 servings

INGREDIENTS

1 teaspoon plus ¼ to ½ cup milk
3 eggs
3 cups gluten-free all-purpose flour
Salt
Freshly ground black pepper
4 cube steaks
2 tablespoons vegetable oil, for frying
Mashed potatoes, for serving

1. Beat 1 teaspoon of the milk and the three eggs together in a medium bowl. Place the gluten-free flour in a separate medium bowl, and add salt and pepper to taste if not using pre-seasoned flour.

2. Allow each cube steak to soak in the egg mixture for at least 10 minutes. Transfer the steaks to the flour mixture and coat them liberally on all sides.

3. In a large skillet over medium-high heat, heat the vegetable oil. Turn heat down to medium, and transfer the coated steaks to the skillet.

4. Cook the steaks until they are dark and crispy—5 to 7 minutes—then flip them over to cook the other side. Remove the steaks from the pan and place them on a paper towel–lined plate to remove excess oil. Keep any remaining cooking oil and meat drippings in the skillet.

5. Reduce the heat to low and whisk the remaining milk slowly into the oil and drippings, alternating with 1 cup of the remaining flour mixture. Whisk continuously and add more milk and flour to the gravy if necessary to maintain the desired consistency. Continue cooking until the gravy has thickened.

6. Serve the steaks with (naturally gluten-free!) mashed potatoes and smother it all with the gluten-free gravy while it's still hot.

. . . .

Cowboy Crêpe

I made an amazing discovery while I was in Paris. Apparently buckwheat crêpes are traditional in some neighborhoods. Which means gluten-free crêpes actually exist. Huzzah!

When I started experimenting, however, I realized that I much preferred a crêpe made from all-purpose gluten-free flour rather than buckwheat. And I really prefer a crêpe with jalapeño bacon and sharp cheddar. Voilà! The cowboy crêpe was born, for the best European/American combo since French fries.

Prep time: 10 minutes + 1 hour rest time **Cook time:** 3 minutes per crêpe
Makes: 10 crêpes

INGREDIENTS

6 strips of uncooked bacon
1 tablespoon finely diced jalapeño pepper
6 eggs
3 cups milk
2 tablespoons butter, melted
1 cup all-purpose gluten-free flour
¼ teaspoon xanthan gum
5 tablespoons butter, for the pan
1 cup grated sharp cheddar

1. Place bacon strips in a large bowl and cover with diced jalapeño. Allow to rest for an hour. Discard the jalapeño.

2. Cook the bacon in a skillet over medium-high heat until crisp. Transfer the bacon to a paper towel–lined plate to remove excess fat. Allow the bacon to cool, then crumble it into small pieces. Set aside.

3. Mix the eggs, milk, and melted butter together in a medium bowl. Slowly whisk in the gluten-free flour and xanthan gum until the mixture is smooth.

4. Melt a half-tablespoon of butter in a lightweight 8-inch skillet or crêpe pan over medium-high heat. Pour ½ cup of batter into the skillet and immediately swirl the pan so the batter coats the entire pan evenly.

5. Cook the crêpe until the edges begin to dry and curl, then flip it over to cook the other side for about 30 seconds, or until golden brown. (If your pan is not lightweight enough, use a large spatula to flip.)

6. Remove the crêpe from the pan and transfer it to a plate. Repeat the process with the remaining batter, wiping out the pan and melting another half-tablespoon of butter before adding the batter each time.

7. Divide the jalapeño bacon and cheddar evenly among the finished crêpes, roll, and serve.

. . . .

Fried Chicken & Waffles

Let's talk about missed opportunities. As in, I lived in Los Angeles for almost a year before I was diagnosed with celiac, and not once did I enjoy a meal at Roscoe's House of Chicken and Waffles. That's just craziness, which is why I now whip up gluten-free variations of both in my own home and pretend my husband is taking my order.

You can also buy a pancake and waffle mix to get this delicious combo onto your plate and into your belly even faster.

Prep time: 20 minutes **Cook time:** 25 minutes

Makes: 8 servings

INGREDIENTS

For the Fried Chicken:

1 chicken, cut into pieces

Salt

Freshly ground black pepper, to taste

2 to 3 cups buttermilk (enough to cover)

3 cups all-purpose gluten-free flour (I use Better Batter Gluten-Free
   Seasoned Flour; see Note)

1 tablespoon salt

1 tablespoon pepper

1 tablespoon paprika

2 teaspoons chili powder

Oil for frying

For the Waffles:

2 cups all-purpose gluten-free flour

1 teaspoon xanthan gum

2 teaspoons baking powder

2 eggs

1½ cups buttermilk

¼ cup vegetable oil, plus more for the pan

1 tablespoon sugar

Maple syrup, for serving

Note: If you're using Better Batter Gluten-Free Seasoned Flour, skip the spices! The batter mix is preseasoned.

1. Make the fried chicken: Season the chicken pieces with salt and pepper to taste, then soak them in the buttermilk for at least two hours.

2. Combine the gluten-free flour, salt, pepper, paprika, and chili powder in a gallon-size zip-top bag. Place the chicken inside the bag, three pieces at a time, seal, and shake the bag to fully coat the chicken pieces. Repeat with the remaining chicken.

3. Heat oil in deep frying pan on medium-high heat. Turn the heat down to medium as you place the chicken in the pan, three to four pieces at a time, leaving plenty of room in the pan to flip chicken.

4. Remove the chicken when its internal temperature reaches at least 165°F, and place the chicken on paper towel–lined plates to remove excess oil.

5. Make the waffles: Coat the waffle iron with a light layer of vegetable oil and heat the iron.

6. In a large mixing bowl, combine the gluten-free flour, xanthan gum, and baking powder, and mix well. In a small bowl, beat the eggs, and add them to the flour mixture. Mix in the buttermilk, oil, and sugar, and set aside.

7. When the waffle iron is hot, scoop ½ cup batter (¼ cup for smaller waffle irons) onto the cooking surface and cook according to the manufacturer's instructions. Continue to make each waffle one at a time until you have used all the batter.

8. Place chicken on top of waffle, drizzle with maple syrup, and serve.

. . . .

Beef Stroganoff over Rice

There's something incredibly filling and comforting about beef Stroganoff, even without the egg noodles. You may not find this version in one of those hip Ukrainian restaurants in Brooklyn, but that's OK because you can't go there anymore.

When you've got a creamy steak with a peppery bite and soft rice to shovel into your mouth, you're satisfying that urge to eat well and hibernate for winter. So you should probably eat this every day for the first three months of your diagnosis because let's face it, "unsatisfied" is going to be your go-to feeling.

Prep time: 10 minutes **Cook time:** 20 minutes
Makes: 4 servings

INGREDIENTS

2 pounds sirloin steak
2 teaspoons salt
1/2 teaspoon pepper
1 tablespoon olive oil
1/2 cup dry sherry
1/4 cup gluten-free beef broth
1/2 cup sour cream
5 cups cooked white rice, for serving

1. Slice the steak into 1/4-inch strips. Season with the salt and pepper.

2. In a medium-size skillet over medium-high heat, heat the olive oil. Add the steak and cook until just brown but not cooked through, about 1 minute per side. Remove from the heat and set the steak aside on a plate.

3. Add the sherry and beef broth to the same skillet and bring it to a boil, stirring once or twice. Allow the mixture to cook for five minutes, then turn the heat to medium.

4. Add the sour cream to the skillet and stir until thoroughly combined with the broth mixture. Transfer the steak and any juices from the plate to the skillet and cook until the meat is cooked through, 3 to 5 minutes.

5. Serve the steak and sauce over rice.

Spaghetti & Turkey Ricotta Meatballs

I used to make these meatballs all the time but just assumed it was a thing of the past when I was first diagnosed. After all, gluten-filled bread crumbs are a given in most meatballs, which sit on top of gluten-laden pasta. Luckily I discovered that corn pasta can be a delightful substitute for the norm, and I was back in action! Also, gluten-free bread crumbs are not at all noticeable in your 'balls.

Prep time: 30 minutes **Cook time:** 1 hour
Makes: 8 servings

INGREDIENTS

For the Meatballs:
2 pounds ground turkey
½ cup gluten-free bread crumbs
½ medium yellow onion, finely chopped
3 cloves garlic, finely chopped
1 large egg
1½ teaspoons fresh oregano, chopped
¼ cup fresh basil, chopped
1½ teaspoons salt
1½ teaspoons ground white pepper
2 tablespoons olive oil
1¾ cup grated Parmesan
¾ cup ricotta

For the Sauce:
24 ounces tomato sauce
2 tablespoons tomato paste
2 teaspoons ground white pepper
6 leaves fresh basil

1 package gluten-free spaghetti

1. Make the meatballs: Preheat the oven to 400°F.

2. In a large bowl, combine the ground turkey, gluten-free bread crumbs, onion, garlic, egg, oregano, basil, salt, 1 teaspoon of the white pepper, the oil, and 1 cup of the Parmesan and mix until completely combined.

3. Roll the turkey mixture into meatballs and place them on a baking sheet. Bake for 25 minutes.

4. Combine the ricotta, the remaining Parmesan, and the remaining white pepper. Set aside.

5. Make the sauce: In a medium saucepan combine the tomato sauce, tomato paste, white pepper, and basil leaves, and simmer for 20 minutes. Remove the basil leaves before serving.

6. Remove the meatballs from the oven, and dollop a spoonful of the ricotta mixture on top of each meatball. Return to oven for 10 minutes more.

7. While the meatballs are cooking, prepare the gluten-free spaghetti as directed on package.

8. Assemble by topping each serving of spaghetti with 2 meatballs and ¼ cup of tomato sauce.

· ·

Italian Meat Loaf

The ultimate comfort food, meat loaf is almost always chock full of bread crumbs as well. This means your comfort will have to come from your own kitchen from now on.

I love giving meat loaf an Italian twist with some Parmesan and pork, because why not? It's awesome. What's not so awesome is trying to find ground pork sausage that does not have gluten. Applegate makes a great Italian sausage, and perhaps your local butcher does too. Always ask about the casing because that's where gluten can hide.

Prep time: 20 minutes **Cook time:** 1 hour
Makes: 10 servings

INGREDIENTS

2 tablespoons olive oil
½ yellow onion, chopped
3 garlic cloves, minced
⅓ cup gluten-free bread crumbs
1 teaspoon thyme
1 teaspoon oregano
1 teaspoon ground white pepper
2 teaspoons salt
1 pound ground gluten-free hot Italian pork sausage
1 pound ground beef
2 eggs
2 tablespoons brown sugar
½ cup tomato sauce
1 teaspoon wheat-free tamari

1. Preheat the oven to 325°F.

2. In medium saucepan over medium heat, heat the oil. Add the onion and garlic and cook until the onion is almost translucent.

3. In the bowl of a food processor, combine the gluten-free bread crumbs, thyme, oregano, white pepper, and salt, and pulse to combine.

4. In a large bowl, combine the gluten-free pork sausage, ground beef, the onion and garlic mixture, and the bread crumb mixture. Mix until thoroughly combined. Add the eggs and mix well.

5. In a small bowl, combine the brown sugar, tomato sauce, and wheat-free tamari.

6. Press the meat mixture evenly into a 10-inch loaf pan and cover with the tomato sauce mixture.

7. Bake for 40 minutes, then test with a meat thermometer for doneness; the temperature should reach 155°F. Cook for another 10 to 15 minutes, if necessary.

. . . .

Spinach Lasagna Cupcakes

If we were being honest with ourselves, we would all admit that everything tastes better in cupcake form. Which is why when I heard some food truck was going around town making lasagna cupcakes, I set about creating a gluten-free option for those of us who need their pasta in handheld cupcake shapes. Which is to say, all of us.

Prep time: 15 minutes **Cook time:** 1½ hours
Makes: 15 cupcakes

INGREDIENTS

1 box gluten-free lasagna noodles
1 pound ground beef
16 ounces tomato sauce
1 teaspoon oregano
Salt
Freshly ground black pepper
1½ cups ricotta
1 cup mozzarella, shredded
½ cup shredded Parmesan, plus more to top
1 egg

3 cups spinach, chopped

Nonstick olive oil cooking spray, for the pan

1. Preheat the oven to 350°F.

2. In a large pot, bring 6 quarts of water to a boil. Cook the gluten-free noodles according to the package directions. (If using "no-boil" noodles, cook for 7 minutes, or until flexible.)

3. Remove the noodles from water, and lay them out on aluminum foil. When cool enough, cut lasagna noodles into thirds.

4. In a large skillet over medium-high heat, brown the ground beef. Drain the fat from the pan, then add the tomato sauce and oregano to the beef and simmer for 8 minutes. Season with salt and pepper to taste.

5. In a medium bowl, mix the ricotta, mozzarella, and ½ cup of the Parmesan. Add the egg and chopped spinach, and mix well. Season with salt and pepper to taste.

6. Spray a 12-well cupcake pan with the nonstick spray. Arrange 2 cooked noodles in each well in a crisscross pattern to cover the bottom and sides of the well. Layer the other ingredients on top of the noodles, starting with the meat sauce, then the spinach-cheese mixture. Repeat until the wells are full, then cover each well with a noodle and top with the remaining Parmesan, distributing it evenly.

7. Bake for 40 minutes. Allow to cool for 10 minutes.

. . . .

Baked Shrimp Etouffée

Cajun food makes an impression. Or maybe that's all the booze you ingested with your boudin. Which is why I still remember an etouffée that had a little extra somethin'-somethin' from my very first trip to New Orleans, which was ages ago.

After experimenting, I do believe the crust atop this shrimp etouffée is spot on with the roux, and the stew, and now a little cheesy crunch. *Laissez les bons temps rouler.*

Prep time: 20 minutes **Cook time:** 35 minutes
Makes: 10 servings

INGREDIENTS

1 tablespoon butter
1 tablespoon olive oil
5 garlic cloves, minced
1 bell pepper, chopped
1 Spanish onion, chopped
2 celery stalks, chopped
¼ cup millet flour
2 cups chicken stock
½ teaspoon sea salt
⅛ teaspoon freshly ground black pepper
1 teaspoon hot sauce
⅛ teaspoon cayenne pepper
⅛ teaspoon paprika
½ teaspoon oregano
1½ pounds shrimp, shelled and deveined
5 cups cooked rice
2 tablespoons gluten-free bread crumbs
1 tablespoon grated Parmesan
Parsley, for garnish

1. Preheat the oven to 350°F.

2. In a cast-iron skillet over medium heat, heat the butter and oil. Add the garlic, pepper, onion, and celery, and cook until soft.

3. Whisk the flour into the onion mixture until well combined. Add ½ cup of the chicken broth and whisk to combine. Gradually add the remaining broth and cook until the mixture has thickened.

4. Add the salt, pepper, hot sauce, cayenne, paprika, and oregano. Stir, reduce the heat to low, and simmer for about 6 minutes. After 6 minutes, add the shrimp and continue cooking for about 4 minutes more, until the shrimp are pink. Do not overcook the shrimp.

5. Remove the mixture from the heat and pour it into a medium bowl. Place the cooked rice in the skillet, and top it with the shrimp mixture.

6. Sprinkle the gluten-free bread crumbs and Parmesan evenly over the shrimp mixture and place the skillet in the oven. Bake until slightly golden brown, 10 to 15 minutes.

7. Remove from the oven, top with the parsley, and serve.

. . . .

Beef Brisket Frito Chili Pie

I used to live in Austin, Texas, and enjoyed the Texas Chili Parlor a little bit too much. Instead of the traditional ground beef and beans, Texas Chili Parlor uses huge chunks of beef in its chili. Dang, it's good. After I moved away I tried to combine a variety of chili recipes to come up with my own facsimile, and this is what I do now.

It's a pretty medium-heat chili, so if you want to step it up a notch you can add crushed red chile pepper flakes, but I think this is pretty amazoids as is. And guess what? Fritos are gluten-free. That's right, Fritos + beef brisket chili + sharp cheddar = gluten-free awesomeness.

Prep time: 15 minutes **Cook time:** 3 hours
Makes: 4 large servings

INGREDIENTS

1 jalapeño pepper

1 tablespoon vegetable oil

2 pounds beef brisket, cut into cubes

1 tablespoon hot sauce

8 ounces tomato sauce

1 shallot, diced

1 clove of garlic, diced

2 gluten-free beef bouillon cubes

6 tablespoons chili powder

4 teaspoons ground cumin

$\frac{1}{2}$ teaspoon salt

$\frac{1}{2}$ teaspoon white pepper

$\frac{1}{2}$ teaspoon cayenne powder

$\frac{1}{4}$ teaspoon oregano

$\frac{1}{8}$ teaspoon crushed bay leaf

1 tablespoon gluten-free cornstarch, if needed

1 large bag Fritos

2 cups shredded sharp cheddar

1. With a small knife, cut a slit in the side of the jalapeño small enough that no seeds are able to escape. Heat the vegetable oil in a Dutch oven over medium heat. Add the brisket and brown on all sides. After all sides are browned, add the hot sauce, tomato sauce, shallot, garlic, gluten-free bouillon cubes, jalapeño, and enough water to cover.

2. Cover and simmer for 45 minutes, stirring occasionally. Add more water if needed. Remove the jalapeño, squeezing its juice into the chili, but discarding the pulp and seeds.

3. Mix together the chili powder, cumin, salt, white pepper, cayenne, oregano, and bay leaf in a small bowl.

4. Add a third of the spice mixture to the chili and continue to cook, covered, for 1 hour. If the chili starts looking too thick, add more water.

5. Add another third of the spice mixture and continue cooking for another 30 minutes, adding water if needed.

6. Add the remaining spices and cook 15 minutes more. If mixture has become too watery, make a slurry of gluten-free cornstarch and 2 tablespoons of water and add it to the chili.

7. Serve the chili warm on top of a cup of Fritos, topped with grated sharp cheddar.

. . . .

Brisket

Hailing from the land of beef, I had no idea that brisket made in this manner was a traditional Jewish dish until I joined the temple. It is, admittedly, much better than throwing that meat on the grill outside the ranch house. Just don't forget that crispy browning comes from the gluten-free flour, chosen people. I make this every Hanukkah to rave reviews, and there's no way anyone can tell it's me-friendly.

Prep time: 10 minutes **Cook time:** 3 to 4 hours
Makes: 16 servings

INGREDIENTS

1 (5-pound) beef brisket
2 teaspoons gluten-free all-purpose flour
2 teaspoons freshly ground black pepper
1/4 cup vegetable oil
6 onions, thickly sliced into rings and separated
2 tablespoons tomato paste
1 1/2 teaspoons kosher salt
2 cloves garlic, roughly chopped
1 carrot, peeled

1. Preheat the oven to 375°F. Dust the brisket very lightly with the gluten-free flour and sprinkle it with 1 teaspoon pepper.

2. Heat the oil in a large Dutch oven. Add the brisket and brown on all sides over medium-high heat until slightly crisp.

3. Transfer the brisket to a large plate. Keeping the heat at medium-high, add the onions to the Dutch oven and cook them in the oil and meat drippings until they are soft and brown, about 15 minutes.

4. Remove the Dutch oven from the heat and place the brisket, along with any juices that have accumulated, on top of the onions. Spread the tomato paste over the brisket liberally. Sprinkle with the remaining pepper and the kosher salt. Add the garlic and carrot and cover the Dutch oven tightly. Place on the middle rack in the oven, and bake for 1½ hours.

5. Remove the Dutch oven and transfer the meat to a carving board. Carve the brisket into ¼-inch-thick slices. Return the slices to the pot, cover, and return to the oven. Cook until the meat is brown and fork-tender, 1½ to 2 hours longer.

6. Remove the Dutch oven and transfer the roast to a heated platter. Serve with slices of the carrot, onions, and the juices from the Dutch oven.

Dessert

Choco Ice Cream Cake

There was no way in hell I was going to give up my mother's choco ice cream dessert, which she always made for me on my birthday. Those dang Oreos make it all gluteny, but luckily there are multiple brands of faux Oreos on the market sans gluten.

Now my daughter wants me to make this cake every year for her birthday. The world is in balance, yet again.

Prep time: 20 minutes **Freeze time:** 2 hours
Makes: 12 servings

INGREDIENTS

½ cup butter
30 gluten-free Oreo-esque cookies
½ gallon vanilla ice cream, softened
⅔ cup sugar
4 ounces semisweet chocolate
1 (14-ounce) can condensed milk
1 teaspoon vanilla extract
1 small container Cool Whip, or 8 ounces whipped cream
½ cup chopped pecans (or other nuts, if preferred)

1. In a saucepan or in the microwave, melt ¼ cup of the butter. Crush the cookies and mix them with the melted butter. Press the mixture into the bottom of a 13-by-9-by-3-inch baking dish or round 5-quart dish.

2. Cover the crushed cookies with softened ice cream. Cover and freeze for at least half an hour.

3. In the top of a double boiler or in a heatproof bowl set over a saucepan of simmering water, slowly melt the remaining ¼ cup butter, sugar, and chocolate. Gradually add the milk and cook, stirring, until the mixture thickens. Stir in the vanilla, then remove from the heat. Allow the sauce to cool.

4. Pour the cooled sauce over the ice cream layer and return the cake to the freezer until set, about an hour.

5. Spread the Cool Whip or whipped cream over the chocolate sauce, and sprinkle with the pecans. Freeze for at least half an hour, until set.

6. Remove the ice cream cake from the freezer at least 10 minutes before serving.

· ·

Double Chocolate Oatmeal Cookies

My childhood friend Denise "Weezer" Rothermel gave me this recipe when we were preteens, and then I co-opted it for myself. Why, yes, I did grow up in a rural environment where people as young as ten swapped recipes. I also believe I entered this in many a county fair, winning ribbons galore. 4-H do or die, people.

Now, however, I have to make sure my oats are gluten-free (as well as the flour). That's one of those weird sneaky foods that can knock the gluten intolerant on her ass. Luckily, Bob's Red Mill makes gluten-free oats in a dedicated facility for all of your oatmeal baking needs.

Prep time: 10 minutes + 1 hour to chill **Cook time:** 12 minutes
Makes: 24 cookies

INGREDIENTS

1 cup vegetable shortening

¾ cup sugar

¾ cup brown sugar

2 eggs

1 teaspoon vanilla extract

1½ cups all-purpose gluten-free flour

¼ teaspoon xanthan gum

1 teaspoon baking soda

¼ cup cocoa powder

1 teaspoon salt

1 teaspoon hot water

2 cups gluten-free oats

1 (12-ounce) package chocolate chips

1. With a hand mixer, cream the shortening and sugars together. Add the eggs, one at a time, blending well after each addition. Add the vanilla.

2. Sift together the gluten-free flour, xanthan gum, baking soda, cocoa powder, and salt. Stir the flour mixture into sugar and egg mixture.

3. Add the hot water, gluten-free oats, and chocolate chips, and mix well to combine. Chill the cookie mixture in the refrigerator, covered, for at least half an hour. Preheat the oven to 350°F while the mixture chills.

4. Drop the chilled cookie dough in spoonfuls onto an ungreased cookie sheet, about ½ inch apart. Bake 10 to 12 minutes, until the edges are crispy.

· ·

Jack's Devil's Food Cake

This is the ultimate dessert in my family. My grandfather used to make this cake every time we visited. That's right, I said grandfather. Granddad Reeves was a Renaissance man ahead of his time: a college football player who knew his way around the kitchen. Once I knew I could make this cake gluten-free, all was right with the world. Also, incidentally, this is how I learned about never eating the gluten-free dough.

Prep time: 10 minutes **Cook time:** 45 minutes
Makes: 16 servings

INGREDIENTS

For the Cake:
½ cup cocoa powder
2 teaspoons baking soda
2½ cups all-purpose gluten-free flour
1 teaspoon xanthan gum
¾ cup vegetable shortening
2 cups sugar
2 eggs
1 cup buttermilk
1 teaspoon vanilla extract

For the Icing:
1 stick butter
4 tablespoons cocoa powder
6 tablespoons milk
3 cups confectioners' sugar
1 cup chopped pecans

1. Preheat the oven to 350°F.

2. Make the cake: Mix the cocoa powder, baking soda, and ½ cup of water together in a small bowl. Set aside. Sift together the gluten-free flour and xanthan gum and set aside.

3. Using a hand mixer, cream the shortening and sugar together. Add the eggs, one at a time, blending well after each addition. Alternate mixing in the buttermilk and the flour mixture, blending well after each addition, until both have been incorporated. Add the vanilla, then add the cocoa mixture and mix well to combine.

4. Grease and flour (using gluten-free flour) a 9-by-13-inch pan baking pan. Pour the batter into the pan, and bake for 40 to 45 minutes, or until a toothpick inserted into the cake comes out clean. Set the cake aside to cool.

5. Make the icing: In a medium saucepan over medium heat, melt the butter. Stir in the cocoa powder and milk and bring the mixture to a boil. Remove the pan from the heat and add the confectioners' sugar, whisking vigorously to combine. Add the pecans and mix, then pour the icing over the cake.

· ·

Italian Cream Cake

One of my new favorites, this moist and delicious cake with cream cheese frosting also used to be my mother's favorite—until, according to the family cookbook, she had to stop making it "because my kids refuse to eat coconut!" Honestly, how dumb was I? I seriously preferred Pepperidge Farm to this, and now I'm shaking my head at myself. Don't make the same mistake. Make this cake.

Prep time: 20 minutes **Cook time:** 30 minutes
Makes: 16 servings

INGREDIENTS

For the Cake:
1 stick butter
½ cup vegetable shortening
2 cups sugar
5 egg yolks
2 cups all-purpose gluten-free flour

½ teaspoon xanthan gum

1 teaspoon baking soda

1 cup buttermilk

1 teaspoon vanilla extract

1½ cups unsweetened coconut flakes

1 cup pecans, chopped

5 egg whites

For the Icing:

½ stick butter, softened

8 ounces cream cheese, softened

3½ cups confectioners' sugar

1 teaspoon vanilla extract

Chopped pecans

1. Make the cake: Preheat the oven to 350°F.

2. Using a hand mixer, cream the butter, shortening, and sugar together in medium bowl. Add the egg yolks and beat well, until the mixture is smooth.

3. In a medium bowl, sift together the flour, xanthan gum, and baking soda. Mix in the butter and sugar mixture, alternating with the buttermilk, until both have been completely incorporated. Add the vanilla. Stir in the coconut and pecans.

4. In a clean bowl with clean beaters on the hand mixer, beat the egg whites until stiff. Gently fold the egg whites into the batter using a spatula.

5. Butter and flour (using gluten-free flour) two 9-inch cake pans. Pour the batter into the prepared pans. Bake for 30 minutes.

6. Make the icing: Using a hand mixer, cream the butter, cream cheese, and confectioners' sugar together until smooth. Add the vanilla and beat until combined.

7. When the cakes are completely cool, remove them from the pans and place one round on a cake platter. Spread between ¼ and ½ inch of icing on top of the round. Place the second round on top of the layer of icing, then use an offset spatula or smooth knife to ice the top and sides of the entire cake. Sprinkle the top with chopped pecans.

. . . .

Hazelnut Chocolate Cake

My cousin Charis is a dietitian. Which means she is a pro at telling you what you should and should not eat. It also means she sent me tons of great recipes when she found out I was in a gluten-free way.

This fresh-ground hazelnut and chocolate number is courtesy of her mother, my aunt Julia, and became a fast favorite in my family. I mean, it's like eating Nutella, with Nutella icing. Can you say no-brainer?

Prep time: 15 minutes **Cook time:** 45 minutes
Makes: 12 servings

INGREDIENTS

1 cup plus 2 tablespoons hazelnuts
6 ounces semisweet chocolate, chopped
½ cup butter
½ teaspoon salt
1 cup sugar
2 eggs
¾ cup Nutella
Strawberries (optional)

1. Preheat the oven to 350°F. Spray a 9-inch springform pan with nonstick cooking spray and line the bottom with wax paper.

2. In the bowl of a food processor, process the hazelnuts to a fine texture. Do not overprocess; the nuts should not be ground into a paste. Set aside.

3. In the top of a double boiler or in a heatproof bowl set over a saucepan of gently simmering water, melt the chocolate and butter. Stir in the salt, and mix until smooth. Add the sugar, mix well to combine, then remove the pan from the heat.

4. In a small bowl, beat one egg, and stir it into the chocolate mixture. Repeat with the second egg. Fold the hazelnuts into the batter, and pour the batter into the prepared pan.

5. Bake for 45 minutes, or until a toothpick inserted into the cake comes out with moist crumbs.

6. Allow the cake to cool in the pan. In a medium saucepan over low heat, warm the Nutella until it reaches a pourable consistency, then pour it over the cake. Serve with strawberries, if desired.

· ·

Stone-Fruit Kuchen

Although I'm more of a fresh fruit type of gal, my little girl came home raving about her CSA (community-supported agriculture) box of goods that was filled with apricots, plums, and peaches. There were so many options, and such huge quantities of stone fruit, that I knew I was going to have to cook them or they would just go to waste.

So this is what magic happened when I took my mother's recipe for kuchen with peaches and gluten-freed it, added in a mix of stone fruit, and served it up. Everyone went crazy for it again and again, and it became the weekly summer treat, courtesy of the CSA.

Prep time: 15 minutes **Cook time:** 40 minutes
Makes: 12 servings

INGREDIENTS

For the Kuchen:

2 peaches

2 nectarines

2 apricots

½ cup butter, melted

¾ cup sugar

1 egg

1 cup sour cream

1½ cups all-purpose gluten-free flour

⅛ teaspoon xanthan gum

¾ teaspoon baking soda

½ teaspoon salt

For the Topping:

¼ cup brown sugar

¼ cup sugar

¼ cup butter, melted

¼ cup all-purpose gluten-free flour

1 teaspoon cinnamon

¼ teaspoon nutmeg

1. Make the kuchen: Preheat the oven to 350°F. Grease a 9-by-13-inch cake pan.

2. Slice the fruit into halves or thirds, depending on their size. Set aside.

3. Cream the butter and sugar together. Mix in the egg and sour cream. Add the gluten-free flour, xanthan gum, baking soda, and salt. Pour the batter into the prepared pan.

4. Make the topping: In a medium bowl, combine the brown sugar, sugar, butter, gluten-free flour, cinnamon, and nutmeg.

5. Sprinkle half of the topping over the batter in the pan, and arrange the sliced fruit on top.

6. Sprinkle the remaining topping over the fruit, and bake for 40 minutes. Serve warm.

. . . .

Peanut Butter Cup Cookies

My friend Jodie used to make the gluten-filled version of this, yet would never give up her recipe. Therefore, I had to wing it when I wanted to create some gluten-free goodness. If I do say so myself, this cookie is an amazing combo of peanut butter and chocolate. Best cookie in the universe? Quite possibly. I know this because I tried this recipe a zillion different ways in order to find perfection.

Here are the tricks: Use full-size Reese's peanut butter cups and splurge on a really fantastic gluten-free flour for this recipe, just to ensure optimum cookie enjoyment. Try Cup4Cup, Better Batter, or King Arthur's.

Prep time: 20 minutes **Cook time:** 17 minutes
Makes: 24 cookies

INGREDIENTS

For the Cookies:
1 cup butter, softened
1 cup sugar
1 cup brown sugar
2 eggs
1 teaspoon vanilla extract
1 cup peanut butter, at room temperature
1 teaspoon baking soda
1 teaspoon salt
3½ cups all-purpose gluten-free flour
1 teaspoon xanthan gum
24 regular-size Reese's Peanut Butter Cups

For the Chocolate Icing:
1 cup semisweet chocolate chips
1 cup unsalted butter, at room temperature
4 cups confectioners' sugar
½ cup milk
¼ teaspoon salt

1. Make the cookies: Preheat the oven to 350°F.

2. In a large bowl, cream together the butter and sugars. Add the eggs and vanilla, and beat well. Mix in the peanut butter. Stir in baking soda, salt, gluten-free flour, and xanthan gum and mix until well incorporated.

3. Roll the dough into 3-inch balls. Place a peanut butter cup in the middle of each ball and then wrap the dough around it, then roll the dough back into a ball.

4. Place 12 balls of dough on a cookie sheet, spaced ½ inch apart. Bake for 17 minutes. Set aside to cool.

5. Make the chocolate icing: In a medium saucepan over low heat, melt the chocolate chips and butter. Remove from the heat, and whisk in the confectioners' sugar, whisking vigorously to avoid lumps.

6. Add the milk and salt to the icing and set aside to cool.

7. Place the cooled frosting in a piping bag fitted with a plain tip (or a zip-top bag with one corner snipped off), and decorate the cookies with chocolate icing stripes.

Chess Pie

The first time I made my grandma Faye's chess pie for my California-born husband, he almost went into a sugar coma. Having never been exposed to the joy of a sugar-and-buttermilk pie before, his mind was blown that people actually made and ate this all the time where I came from.

Although Grandma always made her own crust, I've officially decided that a box crust—or better yet, a frozen gluten-free crust—is the way to go with gluten-free pie. As someone who was actually able to make a decent piecrust before my lifestyle switch, I've still never found the perfect recipe for a basic gluten-free piecrust that one could actually roll out without incident. Or at least, a perfect recipe that did not involve multiple gluten-free flours and hours of my time.

What I'm saying is buy a box or buy it frozen, and simply have that unbaked gluten-free piecrust ready for these unbelievably sweet ingredients.

Prep time: 5 minutes **Cook time:** 45 minutes
Makes: 8 servings

INGREDIENTS

¼ pound butter, softened
1¾ cup sugar
3 eggs
1 tablespoon all-purpose gluten-free flour
½ cup buttermilk
1 premade gluten-free piecrust

1. Preheat the oven to 350°F.

2. Using a hand mixer, cream the butter and sugar together until light and fluffy.

3. Beat the eggs in a separate bowl, then add them to the butter–sugar mixture. Add the flour and buttermilk, and mix thoroughly.

4. Pour the mixture into the gluten-free piecrust and bake for 45 minutes, or until the center of the pie does not jiggle.

German Cream Cheese Brownies

Yet another winning recipe from Aunt Loretta. I learned that the "German" in this recipe comes from the brand of chocolate. So I decided to stop throwing coconut all over these and let them stand as is. Coconut or no coconut, these brownies have become my go-to snack for every single trip I take away from home. They travel well, and they satisfy any craving I have that would otherwise lead to me shoving gluten-filled cookies in my mouth.

Prep time: 20 minutes **Cook time:** 40 minutes
Makes: 16 brownies

INGREDIENTS

4 ounces German Sweet Chocolate (alternatively, use 4 ounces semisweet chocolate plus 2 tablespoons sugar)
5 tablespoons butter
3 ounces cream cheese, softened
1 cup sugar
3 eggs
½ cup plus 1 tablespoon all-purpose gluten-free flour
1½ teaspoons vanilla extract
½ teaspoon baking powder
¼ teaspoon salt
¼ teaspoon xanthan gum
¼ teaspoon almond extract
½ cup pecans, chopped

1. Preheat the oven to 350°F. Grease a 9-inch square baking pan.

2. In a medium saucepan over very low heat, melt the chocolate and 3 tablespoons of the butter. Allow the mixture to cool.

3. Beat the remaining butter and cream cheese together, gradually adding ¼ cup of the sugar and beating until light and fluffy.

4. Add 1 egg, 1 tablespoon of the gluten-free flour, and ½ teaspoon of the vanilla to the cream cheese mixture and mix well to combine. Set aside.

5. In a medium bowl, beat the remaining eggs until light and fluffy.

6. Add the remaining sugar, remaining flour, the baking powder, salt, and xanthan gum to eggs. Mix in the cooled chocolate mixture, then add the almond extract and the remaining vanilla. Set 1 cup of the batter aside.

7. Pour the remaining batter into the prepared pan. Pour the cream cheese mixture over the batter. Drop the reserved 1 cup of batter on top, in tablespoons, and swirl it together with the cream cheese layer.

8. Top the batter evenly with chopped pecans. Bake for 40 minutes.

. . . .

Gluten-Free Coconut Macaroons

Every year at Passover my kids are clamoring for macaroons. While many of them are naturally gluten-free, you don't want to get stuck in the bathroom in the middle of Pesach. So whip these up instead!

Prep time: 15 minutes **Cook time:** 20 minutes baking time
Makes: 20 cookies

INGREDIENTS

2 egg whites
Pinch of salt
1 (14-ounce) can sweetened condensed milk
1 ¼ teaspoons vanilla extract
1 (14-ounce) bag sweetened coconut flakes

1. Preheat the oven to 325°F. Line a baking sheet with parchment paper.

2. Combine the egg whites and salt in a clean metal bowl and whisk with an electric mixer until the egg whites form soft peaks.

3. In a separate bowl, combine the condensed milk, vanilla, and coconut.

4. Gently fold the whipped egg whites into the coconut mixture. Place the batter in the refrigerator, covered, for 20 minutes.

5. Drop the chilled batter by the tablespoon onto the prepared baking sheet. Bake for 15 to 20 minutes, or until golden brown.

· ·

Gluten-Free Coffee Shake

Here's the thing about Starbucks: They cannot be trusted. After making my skinny vanilla latte discovery, I realized that buying any special coffee drink puts your gut at risk. Hence, my newfound love of whipping up gluten-free "frappucinos" in my own house! The recipe makes three fraps, so invite two friends over to share.

Prep time: 15 minutes **Mix time:** 3 minutes
Makes: 3 big coffee shakes

INGREDIENTS

2 cups dark-roast coffee, cooled
1½ cups milk
2 tablespoons agave syrup
2 tablespoons vanilla maple agave syrup
1½ cups ice

1. Put these delicious ingredients into a blender and blend until the ice is broken up and the mixture reaches the consistency of a frappucino. Pour into tall glasses and serve!

Cocktails

. . . .

Ginger Lemon Kick

Let's face it, gluteniacs, you need a drink. Also helpful? A drink that soothes that upset stomach. Add ginger to your cocktail, and you can pretend that you're drinking for medical reasons. Which you are.

I prefer to use one of those artisanal ginger sodas for this recipe, rather than ginger beer or ginger ale. But you can substitute either of those beverages if that's what you have on hand. If you're using ginger ale, you can skip the simple syrup.

Makes: 1 fine cocktail

INGREDIENTS

1 ounce vodka
1 ounce fresh squeezed lemon juice
2 ounces ginger soda
½ ounce simple syrup
Ice
Lemon wedge

1. Add the vodka, lemon juice, ginger soda, and simple syrup to a cocktail shaker with 3 ice cubes. Shake until well blended.

2. Pour into a highball glass over ice. Serve with a lemon wedge.

Tamarind Margarita

Every time I go to my favorite Mexican joint in Los Angeles—Loteria Grill—I order a tamarind margarita. And now, I know how to make up this tart plus spicy number in my own house. The trick is finding the tamarind paste or tamarind concentrate. Look in the Indian or Mexican section in the grocery store or buy it online. A delicious tamarind margarita is a very fancy gluten-free way to consume your tequila. Because you deserve better than the average Joe margarita—you do!

Makes: 1 margarita

INGREDIENTS

Chili powder
Sea salt
2 lime wedges
2 ounces tequila
1 ounce fresh-squeezed lime juice
1 ounce Cointreau
½ ounce tamarind paste
½ ounce simple syrup
Ice

1. Mix equal parts chili powder and sea salt together, and place on a small plate. Use a lime wedge to wet the rim of a rocks glass. Dip the rim into the salt-chili powder mixture. Set aside.

2. In a cocktail shaker, combine the tequila, lime juice, Cointreau, tamarind paste, and simple syrup. Shake vigorously until the tamarind paste is fully dissolved.

3. Pour over ice into the prepared glass. Serve with a lime wedge.

Jell-O Shots, Three Ways

Don't you let them kick you out of the tailgating community just because you can't shotgun a beer like you used to. Show up with these whiskey, tequila, and vodka Jell-O shots and no one can accuse you of being "no fun anymore."

This is the basic recipe for Jell-O shots—yes, you totally do need a recipe—and my suggestions of combos include: Raspberry Jell-O + bourbon; Lime Jell-O + tequila; and Lemon Jell-O + vodka. Go to it!

Prep time: 2 minutes **Cook/Cool time:** 2 hours
Makes: 6 shots

INGREDIENTS

3 ounces Jell-O (any flavor)
6 ounces boiling water
6 ounces booze of your choosing

1. Pour the gelatin into a bowl and add the boiling water, stirring until the gelatin is dissolved.

2. Stir in the liquor.

3. Pour the mixture into 6 shot glasses and refrigerate until set, approximately 2 hours.

4. Shoot it!

Chapter Four

WAITER, THERE'S A
Potential Allergen
IN MY SOUP

I t's possible you've read other books about going gluten-free that say something like "Arrive to dinner at least three hours early to inspect the kitchen. If a non-contaminated surface is not available to specially prepare your meal, come prepared with a bucket of bleach and gloves. Get to work." If that's your jam, well, you'll have a very clean and safe kitchen preparing your food, as well as a dining room full of people trying to take your photo with their phones so they can post about you on the Internet. I, however, am not going to advocate that kind of craziness. I firmly believe that you can, and will, have amazing restaurant experiences without resorting to storming the kitchen and pissing off the very people whom you're asking to take special care with your food. It's cool if you've got the cojones to do this—and *please* write me letters telling me how it goes—and it will most definitely alert everyone to your dietary needs. In fact, there are times I wish I had done this exact same thing. However . . .

I also know that a little charm goes a long way. Hell, a little flirting, maybe a little hinting about how waiters refer to you as "Mrs. Moneybags" about town . . . whatever it takes to get attentive service. Don't rule out a low-cut blouse, ladies. OK, that might have just crossed a line. But I'm not here to judge, just to provide helpful suggestions other than "kick some ass, and take some gluten-free names." You may feel the soft blowing of sunshine up your butt when I say it is possible to walk into a new restaurant without an attitude and not wind up in the bowl all night. It just takes a little bit of effort. I do believe I just heard a collective gluten-free groan. From deep inside of me.

Like anyone who cannot sit down at a table and announce, "Chef's choice!" I *hate* the stress of dining out with crazy food restrictions. My enjoyment of food was greatly reduced with this diagnosis, but I've been fighting my way back to normal. Or rather, what was normal for me. I was the gal who considered a date without a meal not even first-base worthy. When I hit a new town, I arrived with a list of restaurants that I must try, at all costs, even if it meant skipping out early on the Louvre. If there was a farm-to-table opening within a twenty-mile radius, I was the customer showing up early and drooling on the free-range chicken with seasonal stuffing. I was a regular Zagat survey filler-outer until I was forced to completely rewire my brain on no gluten. Had Instagram become popular before my diagnosis, I would have been that annoying friend documenting all of her meals for anyone who cares—and all of those who totally do not (read: most of them). Then came the celiac. Stupid celiac.

Now, my goal is to simply have a delicious meal without getting glutened or making anyone in the restaurant hate me. Growing up in Oklahoma means being polite and not complaining even if you've got a shovel planted in the middle of your forehead. Since I take my heritage very seriously, I always do my best to not be a strain on my server's mental health by being a bad customer, and tip as if she/he had just given me a massage. You don't have to go all Great Plains when you dine out, but I do believe it's possible to be clear about your dietary restrictions, without being a total asshole. Not incidentally, if your go-to persona is "asshole" when you dine out, you really need to stay home until your therapist's work is complete.

So tell us, wise lady, how do we keep it together when we're dining out but somewhat terrified? Well, I'm glad you asked!

Fearing restaurants now that you're gluten-free is totally normal. In fact, you *should* have a little bit of fear in you; otherwise you might just play fast and loose with your meal once too often and wind up in the bathroom all night. Which means you're not getting any action. *And no one wants that.* For the sake of your sex life, please read this chapter, and have your sexee read it as well so she/he knows to take your gluten issues seriously. Like, lack-of-sex seriously.

Go-To Gluten-Free Cuisine

When someone decides to become a vegetarian, the advice starts to flow on the best places to go out to eat without meat. The common refrain is to go ethnic, because there are many cultures who do not worship at the church of bacon as we North American types do. You may think this is a good idea for eliminating gluten from your diet as well, but sadly it is not. The major problem is there is not a culture that immediately springs to mind that eschews wheat, barley, or rye. Maybe triticale. You may be thinking, *But April, I haven't noticed a lot of Wonder Bread in my Chinese food*, and you would be right. However, that devil soy sauce ruins any chances you have of going for dim sum ever again, at least until a totally gluten-free Chinese bistro opens up in Portland, Oregon. *And it will.* I hate being the foul-mouthed bearer of this information, when what I really want to do is to empower you to go out there to Kung Pao Palace and eat until your tender belly is full. You should, however, start at your local taco cart instead.

Mexican Food

Here's the great news. You will still be able to eat mucho tacos. Since authentic Mexican food standards include corn, rice, and beans, you could do worse than to try to live on Mexican food for the rest of your life. In fact, I've considered making this my own personal goal (if by "considered," I mean indulging in biweekly homemade nacho parties). Here are the lovely, naturally gluten-free elements that can (and should!) go into your Mexican feast:

- Corn tortillas
- Pinto or black beans
- Cheese!!!!!
- Grilled meats
- Guacamole
- Salsa
- Tamales
- Tortilla chips*

And that, my friends, is one great big pile of yum. Oh, you noticed that *? Here's your tortilla chip warning: There are two ways tortilla chips can go from rad to pooping your pants. One, if your tortilla chips are seasoned with soy sauce (yes, one brand does this); and two, if your tortilla chips are fried in the same oil as gluten. The same thing goes for hard-shell tacos (aka fried corn tortillas). If they share the oil, you are screwed. Again, this is why the taco stand is so awesome because you're getting tacos and chips—no quesadilla in a flour tortilla, no fried flautas, no deep-fried chile rellenos. This is also why I totally didn't panic after being diagnosed with celiac and heading to Mexico a week later for my family vacation. You can eat well in Mexico, and gluten-free. In fact, start planning all of your vacations to Mexico to ensure healthy eating. You're welcome, Tourism Board of Mexico.

With this said, unless you are in control of your beans, guacamole, cheese, and chips, you still have to ask your server about the preparation. Although it may seem ridiculous to add flour to refried beans, I can guarantee you that some crappy chef somewhere has done just that. Another warning: Mexican food is your friend, but its delicious deep-fried, flour-tortilla-loving cousin, Tex-Mex, is totally not. No more chimichangas for you, my fellow gluten-hater. Go ahead and have a good cry; you've earned it.

Who Are the People in Your (Gluten-Free) Neighborhood?

It's a cliché to say that when you face adversity, you find out who your real friends are because it's totally true. Your being gluten-free is either going to be embraced, ignored, or attacked. Sometimes all three at once, if you're at a particularly drunken dinner party. Let's assume you're not being a jerk about your gluten-free needs, or at least if you are it's because you're having to deal with the asshole who is trying to force-feed you Carr's crackers with foie gras. For those of us who are basically nice people and simply trying to be social while still being gluten-free, here are the five types of friends you'll meet at the buffet.

1. The BFF—This guy or gal will greet you with a gluten-free beer and escort you over to the grill where your burger is being cooked separately—along with its gluten-free bun—before the rest of the gluten-filled grub gets it all messy. You must worship this friend and never, ever, ever do anything to lose this gem.

2. The "It's All About Me" Friend—You say "gluten-free," he says, "I have a rash." No matter what, you're not going to get away from him at the dinner table or for the rest of his life now that he knows he has someone to commiserate with whenever he gets a hangnail.

3. The Passive-Aggressive Friend—She says she totally gets it and loves to offer condolences. Yet she somehow forgets you'll wind up bent over the bowl all night when she orders pizza for everyone to celebrate your job promotion.

4. The Aggressive-Aggressive Friend—Whatever you did to this guy, he is NOT over it. As seen by his constant attacks on your "condition." (Quotes are his.) You tell the waiter you can't eat gluten, he laughs and tells the waiter he can't eat broccoli. You can also depend on him to forward you any articles that include "Kim Kardashian" and "gluten" because he's cool like that.

5. The Ex-Friend—I'm sorry to say it's going to happen. You will find yourself blocking calls from at least one jerk who says, "You're no fun anymore" or talks smack about you behind your back. For some reason when people get sick, some people find it incredibly offensive. Don't worry; you really won't miss her and her evil aura. Seriously, this is someone you probably should have gotten rid of as soon as you saw her duck-face profile pic.

All-American

Sure, Americans love their bread. But if you can take your burger protein-style (in a lettuce wrap without the bun), you're totally set. There are also many hot dogs that are gluten-free, and you can also ditch the bun. Most food that can be thrown on a grill is going to be gluten-free, and who has more grill skills than those of us in the good old U.S. of A.? So what I'm saying is eat meat like an NFL linebacker and you'll be totally OK, gluten-wise. I'm not going to get into the other health issues (ahem, heart disease) because we're just talking about gluten right now. Of course, some restaurants like to get fancy with the marinade on their slabs of meat. Probably because they're un-American. Again, soy sauce could be lurking in that liquid flavor, so always ask your server about the ingredients. If they thicken with flour or jazz it up with soy sauce, you cannot have that meat. You can still enjoy the heck out of the baked potato, though. God bless America!

Did you know that when Americans travel abroad, people from other cultures think we smell like cheese? Well, someone told me that so it must be true. I tend to believe it because, as *Borat* showed us, Americans have more cheese at their disposal than the Dutch and Swiss combined. And I believe everything I see at the movies. As I mentioned before, cheese is your friend in its purest form. So eat up, gluten-frees; it's all good. How should you eat it? How about melted on top of a burger with a lettuce wrap? On top of your French fries not cooked in gluten? Yes! How about served with your crudité? Oh, hell yes. Deep-fried? Only if you do it yourself. My point is, cheese and meat can be found in your local bar and grill, and you should eat them.

Vegetarian

And now for something completely different! Although I found it incredibly difficult to maintain a vegetarian diet without shoving pasta in my gullet, if you go to a restaurant that caters to vegetarians, you'll find much more creative options than my own "pasta and cheese—again" meal. Vegetarians get the dietary restriction thing as well, so you'll likely find an attentive chef and wait staff when you start to unload on them about your gluten. One warning: Seitan is all gluten, all the time. Do not enjoy this meat substitute if you do not want to be in massive gut pain. Also, watch out for that soy sauce. Soy sauce, what is your problem?

Indian

Naan aside, you can eat well at an Indian restaurant without gluten. Chicken tikka masala with basmati rice is a fantastic go-to, as are dal, dosas, saag paneer, and a number of other dishes. Of course you've got to watch out for the samosas, those lovely, lovely deep-fried treats. With all of the amazing flavors found in Indian food, you'll be so satisfied with your meal you won't feel like you've been deprived of anything.

Thai

Hooray for rice noodles! Still, you've got to watch out for the soy sauce and the fish sauce, so choose your Thai restaurant wisely. Not unlike dining out on sushi (which is almost perfect, if not for that dang soy), Thai food is only as good as the people serving you, the gluten intolerant. Although pad thai is almost always guaranteed to be a delicious gluten-free option, you must ask your server. Soba noodles are generally safe, but some do cross over into wheat town. Say it with me: Ask your server!

The best thing about enjoying delicious Thai food is that once you've found a favorite restaurant that's safe, you can always satisfy the Asian food jones that Chinese takeout can no longer soothe (a few Chinese restaurants like P.F. Chang's aside—see Resources.)

Seafood

With the exception of some sauces, if you go to a seafood joint you will be in pretty decent shape. A piece of fish is best served in its most natural state, with a splash of butter, some herbs, lemon, and that's about it. A reputable seafood restaurant won't try to cover up its quality fish by adding lots of things to the dish, and instead works to enhance the fish, as is. Which is great for the gluten-free because that usually means very few ingredients, and for the most part, gluten-free. This of course, excludes Red Lobster.

Red Lobster loves to put gluten all over their seafood, but in their defense, they at least have an allergen menu so you know what to steer clear of while dining at the RL. They also have the disclaimer that food prep areas do not allow them to be truly allergen-free. Although this makes me never want to set food in a Red Lobster, you have to realize that this is the reality in most restaurants. Which brings me to the chain vs. indie discussion.

T.G.I. Friday's vs. Chez Panisse: Ultimate Cage-Free Match

As you start looking around for a place to grab your gluten-free dinner, you'll notice that chain restaurants as well as independently owned establishments are both getting more and more into the whole gluten-free dining scene. Although it's fascinating to me that two different styles of restaurant are both getting on the same bandwagon, it can be difficult to figure out which restaurant is going to safely serve you your broccoli and steak.

Chain restaurants become chain restaurants because they've got a formula that is winning across America, and oftentimes, the world. You may hate McDonald's, but wow, a heck of a lot of people do not. With over twenty bazillion sold, those people have won the restaurant race. The problem with a winning formula is that those chain restaurants have to make sure every one of their 15,000 restaurants across the country serves the exact same thing, with the exact same flavor, every single time. Which is also why some chains introduce a gluten-free menu, realize how difficult it is to maintain consistent safe practices, and later pull it. How do these chain restaurants prep this food so it's all the same? Factories, additives, and preservatives. How does one cover up the fact that a pork chop did not come from the farm across the street, slaughtered earlier that day? Bread crumbs, sauces, and other delicious coverings that will totally make you, the gluten intolerant, sick.

This is why I argue for the farm-to-table type restaurants because the food is fresh, generally organic and/or locally sourced, and additive-free. Most locavore chefs pride themselves on food that is not messed with, which is great for you. Most (not all) chefs at the hot local restaurants also pride themselves on their unique food combinations that are mind-blowingly good. As a foodie, I have nothing but appreciation for the "no substitutions" policy, but as a gluten hater, it kind of sucks. Additionally, a small kitchen (or heck, even a big kitchen) that is set up to deliver the diner the ultimate farm-to-table experience is not set up to make sure you, the gluten intolerant, do not get sick. Although I may prefer this type of dining experience, it's absolutely a risk. And while I can tell you stories of being treated incredibly well at my favorite locavore restaurants around the country, I cannot promise you that you won't get glutened. This makes me sad because I really, really, really want you to explore every restaurant possible and not be afraid to stray from The Melting Pot. Yet I would be irresponsible if I didn't point out that a kitchen that is not set up for the allergic could be a dangerous kitchen.

With that said, I totally enjoy these joints where hipster foodies flock and will continue to do so. What, you may ask, do I do to protect myself? Well, gf gang, I talk to the server very politely. I acknowledge that this is not an awesome thing for me to ask of the very talented kitchen staff, and sometimes even apologize. I smile politely; I tip large. And if I get sick, I never go back. It's not perfect, but it's what I'm willing to do and willing to endure so I can still pretend I'm normal. You may not be willing to do the same, and I have mad respect for that position. I'm simply telling you that if you're feeling sad because you'll never get to hang out at the bar of the newest gastro pub with that crazy chef who always wears a tiara, just do it. Just don't do it every day. Also please note that no doctor worth his/her salt would give you this advice. This is what I, a gluten-free girl who loves her food, am saying that I insist on doing to my own body. If you want to guarantee that no gluten enters your body, you must only visit restaurants that are totally safe. (See Resources.)

Now, let's move on to the more flexible, yet potentially more dangerous, chain options. You *will* find a ton of gluten in fast food and chain restaurants, but many of those joints are getting hip to the program and offering gluten-free menus tucked inside the six-page binder. Hooray! Hooray? Don't get too excited about eating gluten-free in the neighborhood just yet.

It *is* very exciting when you stumble upon a gluten-free menu at a restaurant, no matter what that restaurant happens to serve. Like a two-bit floozy, I ran to any restaurant that advertised a gluten-free menu when I was first diagnosed and looking for a good gluten-free time. It was amazing, relaxing, and offered me some comfort just as I had decided I could never leave my own kitchen again. Then I got sick a few times and realized just because the ingredients in a dish do not contain gluten doesn't mean the pot it was cooked in, the plate it was served on, or the counter on which it was chopped were free of gluten. Unless someone tells you specifically that they do that —and some

The Gluten Rebrand

Let's face it: Gluten is not a sexy word. In order to really sell this gluten-free thing, we need to rebrand gluten. After assembling a highly talented marketing team to create a new gluten strategy, I totally ignored them and came up with some new words for gluten on my very own. Try the following in a sentence such as "I'm _____-free!" Or "I can't eat _____ because it makes me poop."

G-bud   Bongwater

Love poison   Thomas

Sharon Stone   Wheaty McWheatsalot

Toppertot   Fahrvergnügen

Squish

places do (again, see Resources)—you have to ask about the prep and stress that you can't have gluten. Not even a taste.

You're getting the picture, aren't you? You've got to speak up and check up in order to eat safely about town. As a fairly recently diagnosed celiac, I absolutely hate doing this even as I cheerlead you on to doing that exact thing. So much so I turned to Alicia Woodward, the editor in chief of *Living Without* magazine, to ask for some advice on dining out gluten-free. Lucky for me, Woodward is also a psychotherapist, so she nailed it for me. "I'd love to talk to you in five years," she said when I told her I had zero desire to challenge the guy on the Chipotle line who did not change his gloves after handling a flour tortilla. Although my argument would be something like "Do you really want to be that person who holds up the lunch rush?" Woodward reminded me that it would be totally appropriate to do something like ask, "Can you make me another one that's clean?" She cheered me on by saying, "They would count that as a learning experience for the server. You've got to be well, and your health is worth fighting for. Maybe that guy at Chipotle needs to be reminded." So I decided to try again because this smart, nice lady told me I could do it. Also, it's about time I served as a good example to you people, rather than a cautionary tale.

You may be wondering how it's possible for someone with so many curse words in her vocabulary to be completely cowed by walking into her local Chipotle and asking the server to change his gloves. I was wondering the same thing as I took a left turn instead of a right outside of my neighborhood and traveled to the Valley instead of my usual joint in Hollywood. You guys, *I went to the Valley because I was too scared to talk to a Hollywood Chipotle employee.* I found myself needing Woodward's psychotherapy right about then.

Here's the difference between eating fast food and sitting down at a restaurant when you're gluten-free. My feeling has been that your wait staff at a restaurant is ready to make you happy. I'm happy when I'm not getting glutened. So even though I don't love the experience of trotting out my special needs at my favorite bistro, I feel like I'm being ridiculous to expect someone to stop what he/she is doing and fix me a clean trio of tacos when fifteen people are in line behind me, hungry, and craving *barbacoa*. This feeling was intensified as I had plenty of time to stare at the assembly line of not one but four employees I was now going to have to ask to change their gloves. That's eight gloves, people. I almost walked out.

Instead, my love for Chipotle guacamole propelled me to the front of the line, where I said to the very nice man, "Hi, I have celiac disease, and I was wondering if you would mind changing your gloves before you make my tacos." When he said, "What?" I almost ran out. Yet I summoned up the courage to say (somewhat inaccurately), "I am allergic to flour tortillas; could you change your gloves before making me hard-shell tacos?" Here's how it went down. I looked over at the cook who was watching the young man change his gloves. I swear I saw a snicker. The server filled me up with pintos, and I made the decision that I was just going to have to live with three other people getting gluten all over my food because I was not asking *one more person* to change his gloves. Then something magical happened right there in the Studio City Chipotle. With just a whisper, the young man convinced the second server to trade places as he moved my tacos down the line. Then another server was displaced as he shepherded my tacos all the way to the end of the line, even covering my to-go order with foil before the last lady in line could put her gluteny little hands all over it. As I thanked this man profusely, while the rest of his team was looking at him like he was nuts, I could not believe my luck. Apparently that was one employee who needed no reminders of training, unlike me. Naturally I filled up the tip jar, and then realized, "Oh my god, I'm such a jerk. I never tip at Chipotle." I may never go back to that particular Chipotle out of embarrassment, but it will not be out of fear that they don't know what they're doing in that joint. I took home a pair of balls along with those delicious tacos. Yes. I. Did.

I know I'm a huge weenie, but here's the thing. As Woodward reminded me, every person who is gluten intolerant, celiac, has a wheat allergy, or is just sensitive lies in a different place on the symptom spectrum. The severity of your symptoms will most likely inform how adamant you are when you talk to people in the food-service industry about your meal. Some of you poor people will get knocked out for a week and have to miss work if you ingest gluten. There are celiacs who, after even breathing in flour in the air, suffer neurological symptoms for the long term. Then there are people like me who deal with an expulsion of their insides for a day or three, and then get on with it. Who do you think is going to be more likely to frog march that server into the bathroom and make him/her remove those gloves, scrub down with hot water, then come back and try again? Technically, we all should (perhaps in a more gentle manner than described) because ingesting gluten hurts your insides, even if you don't have an immediate outward symptom. The fact is, the only way to stay healthy when you have celiac disease is to be completely adamant about not eating gluten. This means you have to speak up, clearly and loudly, when necessary. I may not be great at it now, but I'm getting there. You should make it your goal to be much, much better than me.

One way people try to negotiate a restaurant successfully is to exaggerate their symptoms when dining out, just to make sure the staff is taking their dietary needs seriously. I would never tell someone I might go into anaphylactic shock if I get even a speck of gluten on my plate, but if you've got the nerves of steel to do it, well, I won't stop you. Your spouse and/or friends may be another story. Let's not forgot those who have to dine with us, shall we?

This is where I praise my husband for always having my back. On those nights out when all I want to do is drain my cocktail and dig into a plate full of yum, he'll make sure the restaurant staff understands that I'm "special." Sure, maybe he's doing it to make fun of me, but I'm also pretty sure he's doing it because a) he loves me and b) after a night out he doesn't want to be the only one able to wake up and take care of the children the next morning. You need one of those advocates for your health. Get one, and dining out will become less strenuous because you can spread the information-sharing responsibilities around a bit.

Let's Talk About Cross-Contamination, Restaurant Edition

A girl's gotta eat. So although cross-contamination might not destroy you in the moment, it can cause damage to your gut even if you're not feeling explosive in your pants. You'll find out if you are sensitive to cross-contamination in a restaurant in the obvious ways very, very quickly. It might take an endoscopy, however, to discover if that cross-contamination is causing you serious harm in your intestines.

Although you should try to avoid cross-contamination at all costs, if you're dining out at a restaurant that serves gluten, and does not specifically have a policy in place about keeping all prep areas separate, you are at risk for cross-contamination. Do your research before you head out to see if the restaurant has an understanding of gluten and how gluten cross-contamination can happen. You'll find out quickly if the restaurant you want to throw a load of cash at has the first clue about your situation. Yes, even if they offer a gluten-free menu. It works like this: You order the gluten-free pizza. Even if the pizza crust has been kept far away from gluteny surfaces, the toppings may be lolling about with other gluten-filled foods. Even if they use a clean pizza stone or baking tray, maybe the slicer, spatula, or other kitchen tool is working double duty. Say you order a salad; the vegetables could have been cut on a surface where bread was also sliced. Enjoying a hunk of meat with no gluten? Of course you are! Let's just hope it didn't hang out next to the breaded chicken cutlets.

You may think these examples sound extreme. Like, seriously, are you going to get sick because your salad was served with a slice of bread, which the waiter promptly removed and you totally didn't eat the piece of lettuce it was laying across? You might. Gluten is so damn sticky that it can glom onto any surface and then stick onto your pure, gluten-free food. Although I may have been able to get out of a dinner date when gluten was served up by the bucketful with no ill effect, you may not. Also, I wasn't so lucky the second time.

As someone who loves dining out, loves food, and hates being told "no," let me assure you that I do not let this cross-contamination issue keep me from the latest gourmet hot dog restaurant opening. But I have paid for that enthusiasm. If you don't want to put yourself at any risk at all, stick to the safe spots and eat at home. You don't have to be a hero. After all, there are plenty of ways you can accidentally ingest gluten without serving yourself up to a wait staff that is either uneducated or unconcerned.

So When Do I Have to Get Crazy and Demand to See the Kitchen?

Admittedly it takes a lot to get me to put down the fork and leave a restaurant. Like a fat mouse running across my foot, for a totally true example. There comes a time, however, when gluten-free people must turn tail and run. My time went something like this: I was invited to a food event, which will remain nameless. The idea was I would be super impressed by what they had to show me (and other food writers) and go home and sing praises to the awesomeness of the food. Although much food was presented that was delicious and gluten-free, when it came time for us to dine, it was all gluten, all the time. Upon realizing the situation, the man who invited me was mortified. His boss, however, looked at me like I had just taken a dump in the middle of the dining room table. Which I could have done, incidentally, had I taken her advice to "Just eat it anyway." Being the polite celiac I am, I offered a quick and easy solution of my just running out and getting a gluten-free item because you know, I'd totally seen them on the tour. The boss lady was not having it. Quite frankly, my gluten-freeness had greatly offended her, and she was not about to go out of her way (which would have taken, like, one minute) to provide me with food that was safe for me to eat. That's when you have to demand access to the kitchen and hover over your dish every step of the way, or leave. I would suggest leaving.

The sad thing is, this will happen to you. It's only happened to me once with so much rudeness, and then one more time with just total incompetence. I prefer the incompetence, and so should you. At least then you can pity the fool. Your body doesn't know the difference between incompetence and evil, though, so it's just going to feel like crap no matter what. Treat yourself gently, and remember tomorrow is another gluten-free day.

You don't want to eat where anyone—wait staff, chefs, or even the hostess—is hostile. Before you were gluten-free, you could probably navigate a shitty situation like this and call it an off night. Now you've got to abort the mission. Your health is too important to leave in the hands of someone who is already mad at you for simply existing, so get out before you're poisoned.

I wouldn't be doing my job, however, if I did not provide you with other options when your dining out experience goes wrong, and fast.

Instead of leaving in a cloud of misplaced humiliation, why not try these perfectly reasonable options:

- While ordering, go down the entire menu pointing at each option asking, "Does this have gluten in it? What about this one? And this?"
- Announce that you're scouting out the restaurant for your client, Mr. Clooney, who has a horrible, secret gluten allergy.
- Ask for the restaurant's attorney's contact information, "just in case."
- Hand the waiter your "Do Not Resuscitate" order, also "just in case."
- When your dinner is served, take a bite, scream loudly while clutching your throat, and fall to the ground. Repeat.
- Excuse yourself to the restroom when your server brings the check. Stay in there until closing time.
- Or, you know, just leave.

You guys, I really don't want to discourage you to dine out. After all, if you're cooking for yourself all the damn time, those dishes are going to make you lose it faster than massive diarrhea and brain fog ever will. You do have to be vocal, never make assumptions, and be willing to go batshit crazy and/ or leave on the rare (very, very, very rare—I promise!) occasion. But don't worry too much; after all, there's always the booze.

Gluten-Free Booze

In spite of what you may have been told by the Internet, most alcoholic beverages are actually gluten-free. Not beer, except for that gluten-free kind, and not malt liquor. So put away your Zima, and pick up these delightful liquors instead.

- Wine

- Vodka

- Gin

- Scotch

- Rye whiskey

- Bourbon

- Regular whiskey

- Rum (dark and light)

- Vermouth

- Tequila

- Brandy

- Port

- Bitters

- Everclear

- Cider

Additionally, the latest policy on labeling for gluten by the Alcohol and Tobacco Tax and Trade Bureau excludes any alcohol that originally was made with wheat, barley, rye, or triticale but distilled to remove the gluten. Therefore, these items would not be labeled as gluten-free. This covers whiskey, rye, some vodkas, and even a handful of gluten-free beers. Of course, the FDA is still working on their rules, and they may be totally willing to overlook this decision. If someone removed the gluten from my cocktail, that's good enough for my dietitian and me. Bottoms up!

Now as you hustle up to the bar and order your dry gin martini, remember that adding stuff to your drinks is OK, so long as that stuff is not gluten. There aren't a whole lot of foodstuffs hanging out at the bar that contain gluten, but there are a few tricky ones to watch out for when you need to quench that thirst. Here's a list.

- Bar snacks (even nuts—some are covered in a glaze of gluten)

- Flavored liquors—stick to the straight stuff, and flavor with natural juices

- Hard lemonade

- Smirnoff Ice

- Beer cocktails (Michelada, Shandy, Black Velvet)

- Wine coolers

We know you don't really drink wine coolers anymore now that you're not in high school, but just in case, you should know wine coolers totally have gluten. Bartles & Jaymes don't look so innocent anymore, now do they?

Although you may begin to acquire a reputation, know that you can always hang out at a dinner party just drinking booze. Occasionally slipping into the bathroom to eat almonds out of your bag is totally appropriate if no one has provided gluten-free food for you. Totally appropriate, and potentially adding to your "reputation."

Here's some good news. There are a few food items that actually taste better when the gluten has been removed. I know! We were totally excited to make this discovery as well. Get ready—here's what you will enjoy even more in its gluten-free form:

Pretzels

Bagel chips

Pizza crust*

Yep, that's it.

*My husband made me add that because he insists gluten-free pizza crust is better than the norm. I totally disagree, but if someone who is able to eat gluten says so, I have to print it.

Chapter Five

WHAT'S
Vegan, Paleo & CrossFit
GOT TO DO WITH IT?

Nothing. But here's the thing. Once you go gluten-free, you get thrown into that whole alternative lifestyle crowd. No, not swingers—which, quite frankly, would be far more welcome than everyone who insists I should give up goat cheese while I'm at it—but the vegans. And on the other end of the spectrum you've got the paleo diet crew. You know, those meat-eating savages who probably pick their teeth with mastodon bones. Elsewhere you've got to keep an eye out for the dairy-free, the nut-free, and the trans-fat free—they're *all* coming after you. Mostly because you shop in the same place now, plus you seem weak from all of that weight loss. I've met more vegans and paleos in the past two years than aspiring actors in Hollywood. I'm not even kidding. As someone who used to turn my nose up at the vegan cupcakes in my local gourmet food shop, I feel I now have to apologize for such snobbery or I am at risk of offending my newfound friends. Also, I probably eat more vegan doughnuts than the average gal, so I've finally learned the lesson from my childhood about "Try it, you'll like it!" I would, however, like to make a point about not giving in to the trend. Any trend.

As the number of vegans and paleos grow and grow, so do the gluten-free. We all have our reasons for hopping on one or more of these wagon trains, and for the most part people know what they're doing and go into it with the best of intentions. Or are forced into it and have zero intention of keeping with it as soon as someone tells them they don't have to eat brown rice crackers anymore. It is not to you people that I address the forthcoming rant. It's you other people: the diet hoppers. (Please prepare your "You're just jealous" retort, 'cuz it is totally true. I'm hella jealous.)

Giving up gluten because you have to is far different than choosing a fad diet because you want to tweet, Instagram, and Facebook your fantastic dinner that's made from monks who don't even have a word for gluten. Although I take no issue with fad dieters per se, I do resent being lumped in with people who are "trying to give up gluten" simply because *I don't want to be here.* Sure, I make jokes about gluten-free this, and pooping that, but you know what? I wish I'd never heard of celiac. There, I said it.

I'm not on a noble mission here with this gluten-free business, I'm just trying not to cry when I think about all the things I cannot have anymore. I'm trying not to freak out about the increased possibility of other random diseases and my chances of having to also give up dairy. Every day that I'm not totally locked up in my house with a fully stocked pantry and refrigerator is a day that I risk getting sick and/or going hungry. In spite of what I might say in this book and in mixed company, this is not nearly as fun as a barrel of monkeys. I don't think it's cool when I have to announce that I'm gluten-free; in fact, I feel like a total jackass 99.9 percent of the time. You guys, there are people I've met since my diagnosis who simply refer to me as "Gluten." I tell ya, I'd much rather be called "Toots" because that name implies that I'm just a lady of questionable character, rather than one with special dietary needs. Most people find that more acceptable.

You know how you can tell the difference between someone who does something for health reasons rather than hipster reasons? Those of us who have to restrict our diet announce it with shame rather than glee. I just wish waiters, casual acquaintances, and judgmental relatives could tell the difference.

Going gluten-free is not a way for me to lose weight, or a way for me to lord my food superiority over others, and especially not a way for me to look hip. If that's what it is for you—good for you, I guess. It's totally true that you're helping to spread awareness, if not annoyance, and for that I suppose I should thank you. So thanks for letting everyone know that there's something called a "gluten-free diet." Your work is done here; now please move on.

Please note that I am not suggesting those of you who go gluten-free because you truly believe it will help with physical ailments are of the "trendy" type. Anyone here who is giving up gluten out of concern for their health is firmly in the same boat as the diagnosed celiac: the gluten-free boat on its way to Deprivation Island. Let's meet those others already on the island, shall we? Perhaps they'll share their coconuts.

I bring up the vegans and the paleos because in spite of their dramatic differences between each other, we gluten-free types have a kinship with both. When you meet them, you will both smile and look each other in the eye and *just know*. There is something extremely appealing about these other people who bug the hell out of friends planning dinner parties, and you're going to enjoy the company of the similarly fated. You should still beware of joining any food cults, but hey, these are (mostly) nice people. The extremely food conscious honestly feel if you're going g-free, why not cut out other potential allergens or irritants and be as healthy as you can be. I get it. I aspire to be one of those people, but I'm weak and from Oklahoma. Also, I'm miserable enough without the gluten, thank you very much. Although I'm not there yet, let's say you are. I've got some tips and tricks for convincing yourself that you're still a "normal" even if you go far afield.

"But April," you say, "paleo is all about chowing down on meat, and vegans are all about being nice to animals. How could these both be bedfellows to the gluten intolerant? And what is this CrossFit you talk of as well?" I know you're all very excited about CrossFit, but let's talk food for a minute. First up, the vegan crowd.

Meet the Vegans

Vegans follow a diet that is absent of any animal products. It's not just meat (which would be vegetarian), it's also dairy. Some vegans choose this as a lifestyle rather than simply a healthy way to eat and go all the way by not wearing or using any animal products (aka leather) as well. It truly is a moral path for those who believe animals have no place being used for human consumption, in any fashion. Nope, not even butter. Some people—and again, I *wish* I were those people—simply want to feel like their conscience is clear when they eat a cookie. They make the choice to eat vegan because it's also cruelty-free. Absolutely no animals are involved in that dinner. Others just want to get on with the milking of the cow. No judgments on which category you find yourself in on any given day.

Although gluten is certainly animal-free, and therefore a staple of the vegan diet, you frequently find gluten-free and dairy-free lumped together, and almost always the "vegan" label gets tagged on because it is, in fact, a vegan product. You will find these products quite a lot because you're heading to a health food–type store to buy your wacky gluten-free flours, and these folks specialize in nontraditional (read: non-Western, non–Dairy Queen–like) foods. You know it's going to be challenging to get millet flour in your local Piggly Wiggly, but the Whole Foods will have both an organic and nonorganic version of that stuff. Shopping at stores where people are hyperconscious about the ingredients in every bit of your food is where you're at now. You may not like it, but you're going to have to learn to embrace your otherness, and try not to judge those around you who think dairy is an even more horrible enemy than the devil gluten.

You may also be shocked to discover the dairy has been removed from your store-bought bread and cookies along with the gluten. These processed gluten-free foods sometimes take the trip all the way to vegan. My guess is makers decide once you make the effort and spend the cash to remove all gluten from your food processing, why not remove dairy as well? Additionally the demand for gluten-free is not as large as gluten-filled, just as the demand for dairy-free is not as large as those who demand the dairy. So you can increase your audience by preparing food for two dietary types, with only one product. Makes sense from a production point of view and is super helpful for those people who go all gluten- and dairy-free at the same time.

Personally I'd love some butter in my gluten-free cake, but I get why this is common practice. I'm also guessing the lactose intolerant and vegans miss their normal flour and are getting a bit tired of that chickpea imposter as well. Once we're all chowing down on vegan, gluten-free doughnuts, however, we sing "Kumbaya" in harmony and go about the business of not throwing up our tasty treats. It's a really powerful bonding experience that can be had in non-traditional bakeries all across North America.

There's one more thing about the gluten intolerant and vegan connection that I'm loath to mention. Apparently many of us tend to develop a little dairy problem in tandem with our gluten problem. I'm pretending I never heard that, but some poor souls are just incredibly unlucky. Also, dairy can be difficult to digest (again, lalalala, I can't *hear* you!), so once you're all jacked up on the inside, cooling it on the dairy might be a good idea.

Even though I pretend to ignore any negativity about my milk products, I do like to pay attention to that dairy-free advice about once a quarter. Which is why I happen to have a few amazing gluten-free and diary-free recipes up my sleeve! Since we may as well skip the meat,

I just call these recipes "vegan" and pretend I'm one of those. Why not? I pretended to be goth in college, and that was awesome.

Try these gluten-free, vegan, delicious recipes to sooth your aching belly, and conscience.

Deep-Fried Broccoli & Black Bean Sauce, à la No. 7

I used to live right down the street from my favorite Brooklyn restaurant, No. 7. I was actually thankful we moved after I was diagnosed with celiac because I would cry thinking about how I would never again enjoy their amazing deep-fried broccoli with bean sauce. Then I woke up and realized I could make it my own damn self. Voilà!

You do need a deep fryer to make this recipe a success, but if you don't have one you can always grab your deepest skillet, fill it up with vegetable oil, and turn the broccoli until it's cooked on all sides. Again, if you use a seasoned all-purpose gluten-free flour, then you can skip the salt, pepper, and coriander.

Prep time: 20 minutes **Cook time:** 35 minutes
Makes: 4 servings

INGREDIENTS

For the Bean Sauce:
1 tablespoon olive oil
2 cloves garlic, minced
1 shallot, minced
⅛ cup white wine
⅛ cup sherry
1½ cups black beans
1 cup vegetable broth
2 teaspoons hot sauce
1 teaspoon sea salt
1 teaspoon pepper

For the Broccoli:
1 teaspoon hot sauce
1 teaspoon fine sea salt

2 teaspoons black pepper
1 teaspoon ground coriander
2 cups all-purpose gluten-free flour
1 head broccoli
6 cups vegetable oil, for frying

1. Make the bean sauce: In a Dutch oven over medium heat, heat the oil. Add the garlic and shallot and sauté until translucent.

2. Add the wine, sherry, beans, and broth, and simmer for 10 minutes. Remove from the heat.

3. Using an immersion blender, blend the mixture until smooth. (Be careful! It's hot.) Return the Dutch oven to the stove, reduce the heat to medium-low, and add the hot sauce, salt, and pepper. Cook until thick, about 15 minutes.

4. Remove the bean sauce from the heat and set aside.

5. Make the broccoli: Combine ½ cup of water, the hot sauce, salt, pepper, coriander, and gluten-free flour, and mix well. Completely submerge the entire head of broccoli in the batter. Allow the broccoli to sit in the batter for at least 10 minutes, turning it twice, until all of the florets are coated from stem to flower.

6. Place the oil in a deep fryer and bring to temperature.

7. Completely submerge the broccoli in the oil and fry until a crust forms, 7 to 10 minutes.

8. Remove the broccoli from the oil with tongs, and place it on a paper towel–lined plate to soak up excess oil. Serve immediately, with the black bean sauce on the side.

Pecan Sandies

One of the first recipes I mastered as a young 4-H-er, this recipe is in my family cookbook under "April." Woo-hoo! I made it into the family recipe book. It was relatively easy to veganify this recipe because no eggs are required. It still turns out to be a delicious, light, sugary mess of a cookie.

Prep time: 10 minutes + 4 hours chilling time **Cook time:** 20 minutes
Makes: 25 cookies

INGREDIENTS

1 cup (2 sticks) Earth Balance Vegan Butter
1/3 cup sugar
2 1/2 teaspoons vanilla extract
2 cups all-purpose gluten-free flour
1 cup pecans, finely chopped
1/3 cup confectioners' sugar

1. Using a hand mixer, cream the Earth Balance and sugar together in a medium bowl. Scrape down the sides of the bowl, and add 2 teaspoons of water and the vanilla.

2. Beat in the gluten-free flour. Scrape down the sides of the bowl again and add the pecans. Stir to combine.

3. Cover the bowl with plastic wrap and place in the refrigerator for 4 hours.

4. Preheat the oven to 325°F. Roll the dough into 1 1/2-inch balls and place them on an ungreased cookie sheet, 1/2 inch apart.

5. Bake for 20 minutes. Allow the cookies to cool slightly, then roll them in the confectioners' sugar.

Spicy Chocolate Chip Coconut Ice Cream

Believe it or not, vegans can totally enjoy ice cream. After some experimentation, I discovered that coconut milk gives the richest texture when making vegan ice cream. For this recipe, I also use Theo chipotle spice drinking chocolate, because it is vegan and, quite frankly, amazing.

If you have an ice cream machine, you can easily whip up vegan ice cream whenever you like. I highly recommend that you do.

Makes: 12 servings

INGREDIENTS

2 (14-ounce) cans coconut milk
2/3 cup drinking chocolate with chocolate chunks
1/3 cup sugar
1 teaspoon vanilla extract
1/4 teaspoon sea salt

1. In a medium bowl, whisk all the ingredients together. Transfer the mixture to an ice cream maker, and follow the manufacturer's directions to process it into an ice cream.

2. Transfer the ice cream to a sealable, freezer-safe bowl.

· ·

Versatile Quinoa Salad

You didn't think you were getting out of here without a quinoa recipe, did you? Let's face it, quinoa is your new best friend if you're vegan, or just gluten-free. If you have this salad-like dish in your back pocket, you will never be hungry, and you will always feel superior for knowing how to make quinoa a dozen different ways.

Although we like to go with kale, lentils, and shallot, you can add whatever you like to the mix. Corn, red onion, and quinoa are totally delicious, as is broccoli and quinoa with a lemon dressing. Here's my family's go-to quinoa salad; please make it your own.

Prep time: 15 minutes **Cook time:** 20 minutes
Makes: 10 servings

INGREDIENTS

For the Quinoa:
1 cup quinoa
2 tablespoons olive oil
1 shallot, chopped
1 garlic clove, minced
1 head kale, deveined and roughly chopped
2 cups cooked lentils
Salt
Freshly ground black pepper

For the Dressing:
2 tablespoons wheat-free tamari
1 tablespoon sesame oil
4 tablespoons orange juice
1 tablespoon rice wine vinegar
Garlic clove, smashed, skin discarded
Salt
Freshly ground black pepper

3 green onions, finely chopped

1. Bring 1½ cups of water to a boil in a medium saucepan. Add the quinoa and cook, covered, over low heat for 10 to 15 minutes, or until the water has been absorbed. Set aside.

2. In a medium saucepan over medium heat, heat the olive oil. Add the shallot and garlic and sauté until translucent. Add the kale and cook until tender, about 3 minutes.

3. Add the quinoa and lentils to the skillet and heat thoroughly. Remove from the heat and season with salt and pepper to taste.

4. Make the dressing: In a cruet or mason jar with a lid, combine the dressing ingredients and shake well. Season with salt and pepper to taste.

5. Transfer the quinoa mixture to a serving bowl and top with green onions and dressing.

What Up, Paleo?

Perhaps you're more of a carnivorous trendy type. Then the paleo diet is totally for you. This ancient style of eating is less Captain Caveman and more based on evolution. After all, people's guts were probably a bit shocked at that whole agricultural revolution thing when food started appearing all ground up from plants that were considered "weeds" before. Hell, my gut is shocked every time I drink that POM juice. Although going vegan may seem to eliminate foods from the diet, paleo is more about a very specific list of approved foods going down your gullet. Foods such as grass-fed meat, fresh fruits and vegetables, nuts, and seafood are on the list. Anything processed, such as grains (gluten!), refined sugars, certain vegetable oils, beans, potatoes, and my good friend—dairy—is forbidden. Wow, trendy people really love to hate on dairy, don't they? Poor dairy.

To follow a strict paleo diet, you only eat the foods that would (probably) have been available during the Paleolithic era. Removing grains, refined and processed foods, and dairy is to eat like our ancestors instead of forcing our bodies to adapt to our other, more recent ancestors who learned how to mess with things. I'm halfway between buying this hook, line, and sinker, and between wondering what good we are, as humans, if we don't adapt. Still, I know people who swear by this, and their physicals every year back it up.

Like any movement, different leaders of paleo eating have different theories. Some say you should only eat lean meats because today's meats are much more fatty than those days of yore. Others say to eat that meat fat because it's not dairy fat, and therefore good for you. Some even say tubers like potatoes are totally cool. You will see on the thousands of websites that have cropped up that paleo can be stretched to include things like gluten-free, dairy-free chocolate chips and almond flour. I think we can be pretty confident that cavemen and women weren't enjoying chocolate chip cookies, but hey, *we've evolved.*

My takeaway from trying paleo is this: Don't eat processed foods. When you eat meat, make sure it's grass-fed and organic. Yes, there is a bit more to it—like the potato and bean thing—but if you find yourself confused by the fact that you can't eat rice yet you can drink agave syrup, keep it simple. Although here's the biggest bummer about eating paleo: You can say goodbye to taco night.

Who's hungry for some meat? Right this way to paleo dining. Remember, any meat should be grass-fed, antibiotic-free, and organic. Go organic on fruits and vegetables as well, if possible. Eat up, you Neanderthals.

Pistachio Pesto-Stuffed Pork Chop

Nothing says old school like fancy pesto. Stuff your gob with this delight, and bask in the praise of the meat-eating foodies.

Prep time: 10 minutes **Cook time:** 45 minutes
Makes: 2 pork chops

INGREDIENTS

2 organic pork chops, 1½ inch thick

1 cup plus 1 tablespoon olive oil, divided
½ cup pistachios, shelled
5 garlic cloves
3 cups basil, roughly chopped
½ teaspoon sea salt
1 teaspoon black peppercorns

1. Preheat the oven to 350°F. With a sharp knife, cut each pork chop in half horizontally, but stop 1 inch away from end, creating a pouch in the pork chop.

2. In a skillet over medium heat, heat 1 tablespoon of the olive oil. Brown the pork chops for a minute or two on each side. Set aside.

3. In a mortar and pestle or the bowl of a food processer, combine the pistachios, garlic, basil, salt, and pepper. Beat or process until well combined but not ground into a paste. Transfer the mixture to a bowl, add the remaining olive oil, and mix well.

4. Using a spoon, stuff each pork chop with the pesto mixture. Transfer the pork chops to a baking sheet, and bake for 35 minutes.

5. Turn on the broiler, then allow pork chops to broil for 5 more minutes. Remove from oven and serve.

· ·

Coconut Oil-Roasted Chicken & Spring Vegetables

If you're truly committed to paleo, you'll just grab a free-range organic chicken and bite into its neck. But this way is much, much tastier. It's also true that we all need to know how to roast a chicken. You can make that roasted chicken into several meals, and not feel panicky about the lack of gluten-free food in your house. Go, chicken!

Prep time: 15 minutes **Cook time:** 90 minutes
Makes: 8 servings

INGREDIENTS

1 (5-pound) organic roasting chicken
Coconut oil
6 garlic cloves
1 lemon, quartered
3 cups organic chicken stock
1 onion, chopped
2 bulbs of fennel, chopped
4 carrots, quartered
1 bunch asparagus, ends trimmed
Salt
Freshly ground black pepper

1. Preheat the oven to 400°F.

2. Coat chicken skin, on top as well as underneath, with coconut oil. Dice 3 cloves of garlic and distribute the diced garlic underneath the chicken skin. Place the remaining whole garlic cloves and quartered lemon inside the chicken cavity. Pour the chicken stock into a roasting pan and cover the bottom of the pan with the chopped onion. Place the chicken in the pan.

3. Roast the chicken for about 90 minutes, flipping it upside down halfway through the cooking time. Baste the chicken periodically with chicken stock. Add water to the pan if necessary, to keep it from scorching.

4. Place the fennel, carrots, and asparagus on a large baking sheet and cover with 1½ tablespoons of coconut oil. Season lightly with salt and pepper. Add a splash of chicken stock for flavor, if desired. Place the vegetables in the oven with the chicken and roast for 40 minutes.

5. Using a meat thermometer, check the internal temperature of the chicken; the chicken is done cooking when the temperature has reached 165°F.

6. Allow the chicken to rest for 10 minutes, then serve with the roasted vegetables

. . . .

Almond Coconut Bar

Thank god for honey! It's one of the approved sweet things a paleo person can eat (in moderation), so you should throw that all over your treats. Although I'm pretty confident the men and women of the Paleolithic era did not enjoy these bars after their workout, you can!

Prep time: 10 minutes **Cook time:** 20 minutes
Makes: 8 bars

INGREDIENTS

1 cup almonds, chopped or slivered
½ cup coconut flakes
¼ cup almond butter
¼ cup organic honey

1. Preheat the oven to 400°F.

2. In a medium bowl, combine the ingredients and mix until completely moistened. Pour the mixture into a wax paper–lined 6-by-6-inch square pan. Using another piece of wax paper, flatten the mixture to a thickness of ½ inch. Remove the top layer of wax paper when mixture is evenly distributed in pan.

3. Bake for 20 minutes. Remove from oven and allow to cool for at least 20 minutes before slicing into 8 bars.

Here's the bottom line on trends: I don't know which diet is going to work better for your body. And if you're just trying to be trendy, maybe you should talk to a nutritionist and/or therapist about what your body and mind need, rather than simply grabbing onto the latest thing Miley Cyrus tweeted. There is nothing wrong with choosing an alternative way of eating, and if you're going for a lifestyle change for the better, these two diets are certainly not bad. Some would argue they are two of the healthiest ways to eat, in fact. How to decide which way to go? Veganism has that whole "we don't hurt animals" thing going for it, which is quite adorable. Yet the paleo people are all, like, "It's evolution, dummies." I'm just trying to figure out how to be gluten-free without losing my ever-loving mind, so I'm going to have to put these other decisions on ice. I would, however, very much enjoy a cage match between a vegan and a paleo type in the event that I need to make a decision about either of these diets at some point in the future. That would be the best way to decide, right? Paleos, you'd better watch out because you know those vegans are secretly vicious.

Oh, and that whole CrossFit something is just bonkers. Don't even think about it. It's like fifth-grade gym class for adults who have been honing their competitive dodgeball skills for thirty years. You're going to get hurt, and it's probably not even gluten-free.

Chapter Six

HOLY CRAP, MY KID'S

a Celiac

t's possible you've come here for help because one or more of your off-spring is being forced to go gluten-free. If so, thank you for reading, and I am so, so, so, so sorry. As a mother to one of those "I only eat white" kids, I pray every day that little dude does not develop gluten sensitivity. Because you know what's white? Gluten. It's tough enough for an adult to follow a gluten-free diet, but for a kid who just wants to eat crackers (toddler), or fit in (adolescence), or get his beer bong on (ummm, college? Junior high?), it's a huge drag. You, as the parent, have to be even more of a pain in the ass than usual to make sure your kiddo isn't poisoning himself/herself every single day. This one is tough and completely unfair for your future keg party attendee. Even though in the beginning you can somewhat control your child's food, it will get worse. Negotiating play dates will seem like a wheat-free cakewalk once your child hits prom age. *I know.* Again, please accept my condolences on your bumpy ride into raising this sensitive child without constantly being worried about what he's shoving in his belly. Hey, at least he's not the tree nut kid.

No, it won't be easy, but I can do you a solid and help you raise those kids until they're adults and they finally realize that pooping in their pants is not cute, and so they'd better skip that pizza party. Even though (*sofarthankyougod*) my kids are not in the celiac camp, I still try to feed them mostly gluten-free, which is why I'm becoming an expert in the gluten-free-snacks-for-kids business. I can assure you there is no shortage of packaged gluten-free cookies, crackers, and other goodies marketed directly to kids, some a far better fit into a healthy, gluten-free diet than others. In fact, I *could* make my own kids gluten-free if I wanted to. See, kids? Don't forget this act of generosity when I lose my mind and you're nursing home shopping. Also, don't think I didn't see you waving that bagel behind my back.

I have my own struggles being a gluten-free mom to two gluten-loving kids. Even though I attempt to keep most of the gluten out of my home, I do have to allow for the occasional gluten slippage. Although to be perfectly clear: If it were easier on me to keep a 100 percent gluten-free home, I would do it. In my current situation with two small children—one of whom is picky as all get out, the other of whom has to have a kosher lunch packed every school day—my life is easier filling up their little bellies with bread they will eat rather than complain about. It's not that I like having to step away from their tiny, gluteny hands when they just want a hug after lunch. And do you know how hard it is to avoid a kid with birthday cake all over her face when you're trying to drag her into the car and away from the party that has gone on way too long, and quite frankly has nothing for the gluten-free me to eat or drink? Of course you do because you're at that same indoor play space fighting for your kid's health. Can we just agree that those parties are the freaking *worst*?

The good news is, I've trained my kids to sniff out gluten, and they've become quite protective of their mother. Although this most likely will only last another three to six years before they start using it to their evil advantage (Want to take the car out? Slip Mom some gluten!), right now it's adorable to hear my kiddos ask, "Is there gluten in that?" when we're out. It has the added advantage of making them seem wise beyond their years and/or like totally pretentious California kids. I like to think it's the former. You can do the same for your celiac and gluten-intolerant kids! Kids pick up everything super fast and can adapt in a much smoother fashion than us much older folks. Your gluten-free kid will be standing up for herself in no time and ordering gluten-free off a regular menu. But first, you've got to sit down that little bellyacher and explain what the heck is going on in there, anyway.

Gluten-Free Call & Response

You're not a helicopter parent when your child has a food situation; you're just awesome and ready to protect and defend in all situations. Until your child is old enough to defend himself/herself, as well as curse like a sailor, you're going to have to be the one who talks back to clueless and/or evil people. Here are some scripts you can use! Although I'm totally not responsible for the actions of the people you are about to offend.

WHEN SOMEONE SAYS:
"So what happens when he eats gluten?"

YOU SAY:
"Have you seen *Alien*? Like that, but with more poop."

WHEN SOMEONE SAYS:
"But she won't always have to be gluten-free, right?"

YOU SAY:
"Nope. Only as long as you have to be a condescending asshole."

WHEN SOMEONE SAYS:
"You know, poor people don't have food allergies."

YOU SAY:
"Oh, I'm sorry. I didn't know you were the International Expert on Poor People and How Well Their Autoimmune Systems Function. Forgive me, and please pass the gluten."

WHEN SOMEONE SAYS:
"Don't worry, there's just a light coating of flour on these pork chops."

YOU SAY:
[Withering stare. Later, instruct your child to stink up that person's bathroom.]

The Talk

Even if you discover that gluten hates your baby, at some point that baby will grow up and start in with the "whys," and you will have to explain to your child about what's going on in his body. Finding the right balance between reassuring and instilling the seriousness of the situation is going to be tough. Since I didn't have to do this and instead just said, "Hey, kids, I can't eat gluten," to a room full of disinterested small people, I asked someone who actually knows what she is talking about.

I went back to Alicia Woodward, psychotherapist and *Living Without* magazine editor in chief, to talk about this tricky situation. Woodward agreed that striking a balance between keeping your child safe while encouraging him/her to have a normal, active childhood was a challenge for all parents of celiac and food-allergic kids. After all, screaming, "Don't touch that!!!" at every school get-together is most likely going to have serious and lifelong consequences for your little eater. We don't want our little ones developing eating and anxiety disorders alongside their gluten problem. Woodward advises parents to "stand on the positives." She adds, "These days, there are many positives in the form of wonderful gluten-free products, support groups, summer camps, opportunities for learning and adventure, and restaurant options." True that. One piece of advice from Woodward so totally applies to adults as well: "Keep the pantry stocked with terrific-tasting gluten-free products." It's true. Pirate's Booty and M&Ms can diffuse a meltdown even in your nonallergic kids (and totally allergic adults).

Positivity is super-duper important, of course, but stating the facts about why your kid has to be different is also effective. Woodward stresses that parents should "Talk up the benefits of *feeling better*, being stronger and healthy at last, as well as the benefits of really knowing our bodies and taking good care of this exquisite, elegant machine that carries us through life." It's not a bad way to teach all of our children to think when they think about food. Utilizing the right kind of food is like fuel, and we can all explain eating in a healthy way, rather than an anxiety-inducing manner. Setting a good example is also hugely important, so watch how you talk about food and disease—especially to your gluten-intolerant kid. Focusing on strength instead of weaknesses will go a long way in reassuring your very impressionable child.

Something I would add to the "setting a good example" portion of this advice includes normalizing the disease. You wouldn't disclose that your child has acid reflux upon meeting new people, so don't introduce your child to new friends and immediately announce her celiac disease. Of course you have to inform people if the situation warrants it, but showing your child that she is more than her disease is important too. Take it from someone who gets called "Gluten."

Getting your child truly involved in her eating habits and taking care of her health is also key when discussing the disease. One fab way to do this is to put that kid to work. Since you're totally going to be in the kitchen a heck of a lot more, why not employ some child labor? Woodward advises, "Prepare the wonderful gluten-free alternative grains and flours, and turn an eye to making great recipes from scratch, spending relaxed and pleasant time in the kitchen with your child. Make cooking fun and a taste adventure. This opens a whole new world for your child and teaches great life skills." Personally, I love this idea simply because grating cheese gets old, you guys.

Not unlike adults, it's going to be helpful for your little one to find a support group or even just one friend to talk to about celiac. Woodward suggests that you and your family join a local celiac support group and participate in the fun kids' events. Especially exciting, there are summer camps just for celiac kids (see Resources) where your kids can make lanyards without worrying about some other kid putting gluten all over his pillow at night. Let your child know about these special opportunities, and hop to it. Before you know it, your kid will be eating gluten-free without even thinking about it, and you can relax a little bit as well. Oh, who am I kidding? You're a parent. *You will never relax again.*

Let's tackle this gluten-free dilemma by age, shall we? Trust me, you'll be so stoked to go back to using your panini maker when your gluten-free kid graduates from high school, that empty-nest feeling will be replaced with euphoria. Delicious, gluten-filled euphoria.

The Baby/Toddler Gluten Intolerant

More commonly than you might think, some parents find out their tiniest ones need to go gluten-free early on in the game of life. It is incredibly scary to discover a stomach—or any other—ailment in such a miniature-size person, and after you're finished thanking the maker that it's not something worse, you're going to be cursing that same guy for upending your kitchen, and life. Of course, controlling a baby or toddler diet is dramatically easier than controlling a teenager's, well, anything. But that doesn't mean it's a piece of cake. In fact, *it's the exact opposite of a piece of cake.*

Please don't shoot me when I say nursing an infant for as long as you possibly can is the easiest way to keep a kid gluten-free. It's the one way to remain in total control, and as long as you don't eat gluten, your baby is not getting any gluten either. It's also true that going gluten-free is not at all easy, especially if you yourself have zero symptoms that need to be addressed. That baby time is, however, the last time you'll be able to watch every single nutrient going into your child and act as quality control. So enjoy that! Once your baby is cared for by anyone else—be it a relative, day care, nanny, or that weird lady who lives next door (*Editor's note: Do not let the weird lady next door babysit. DO NOT.*), the chances of your little one consuming gluten dramatically increase. As someone who strongly believes a woman should choose the best way to feed her baby her own damn self, I still have to say if you're breastfeeding or pumping breast milk and it's clear that's all the baby is allowed to consume, your baby will be A-OK. You know, as long as you're not mainlining Krispy Kremes. Which is what you *should* be able to do if you're pregnant, breastfeeding, or even considering doing either of those things.

Alternatively, get on the horn with every formula company in the world. As a working mother myself, I know the value of ready-made, and there will be times that you've gotta have it. Most, if not all, infant formula *is* gluten-free (again, thank the maker), but you have to watch out for any change in recipe by the formula manufacturer and be vigilant about checking. Once you go formula, or day care, or nanny, or weird lady next door, you also have to bear in mind that there are some sneaky old-school people who think giving your baby cereal in her formula is helpful. Or people who think you're a crazy mom who is denying her child. You see where I'm going with this? If you're in charge, you can control the situation. After all, you're the only one manufacturing that boob milk.

As your baby turns into a toddler, you can still maintain control, but you have to start thinking about whether or not you want a gluten-free house. This means you give up the gluten too, and that's not always easy and it's totally sad. Also sad? Your child will never know the joy of joining the Cheerio cult. (But this is great news for your couch cushions and car seats.) So many toddler snack staples contain gluten, it's almost like your kiddos are trained to go on the all-white diet from an early age. In addition to the aforementioned Cheerios, toddlers love anything that looks like a cookie and enjoy to an obscene degree the crunch of a Goldfish cracker and its organic cousin, the Cheddar Bunny. Bagels make many a teething toddler totally chill, as does pasta. You see how it can be difficult to keep a toddler gluten-free?

Luckily all of the above have gluten-free substitutes; they just cost a heck of a lot more. Instead of starting the snacking with flour-based treats, try to ply your toddler with fruit and toddler-friendly vegetables. Yes, I realize what I just said is totally hypocritical given my own kids' penchant for crackers with a side of crackers. But getting your toddler used to eating fruits and vegetables is great for many reasons, not the least of which that you don't have to worry about someone sneaking gluten inside a fresh strawberry.

Rest assured that there are some gluten-free toddler snacks that will satisfy that cracker urge if you can't get them to dine on sugar snap peas and raspberries. I mean, you're not freaking Gisele Bündchen over here. Some of the best naturally (or processed) gluten-free toddler snacks outside of fruits and vegetables include:

- Cheese
- Pirate's Booty
- Rice cakes
- Yogurt
- Fruit leather
- Cereal: Gorilla Munch, Rice Chex, Koala Crisps, and more
- Gluten-free cereal bars

Like so many other parental situations, unfortunately, it's not all about you. Your newest job, in addition to the five million other ones you took on when you acquired that bundle of joy, is educating everyone who comes into contact with your little beggar. Because a kid deprived of Goldfish will beg. You know who is totally susceptible to child beggars? Grandma.

I guarantee you that lady will be the first person to say, "Oh, surely she can have a little." Oh, no she can't, Grandma. Back off. Be prepared to repeat your intense informational sessions, followed by pleas to keep your child safe, followed by threats to anyone who comes into contact with your child—even Grandma. These skills will also come in handy during the truly terrible threes. That's right, I said it. The twos have got *nothing* on the threes. Also, this is excellent preparation for the school years. (Cue ominous music.)

The School Years

Oy. It's happened: Your baby is growing up. Although most of us shed some tears on the first day of kindergarten, it's for existential reasons. As a parent to a kid with gluten issues, you have real reason to cry because there are other lunch boxes out there that are totally dangerous to your little gluten-hater.

There are two ways to battle the coveting of another's lunch: One is to threaten your child and your child's friends within an inch of their little lives about the gluten. The second is to create truly delicious and envy-inducing food for your kid's lunch box so every kid goes home asking if they can also be "gluten-free." It's really your choice which road you take, but please enjoy some of the recipes at the end of this chapter if you decide not to frighten schoolchildren. Additionally here are some great gluten-free lunch box options for bigger kids:

- GF Tortilla Wraps with Cream Cheese & GF Turkey
- Yogurt Squeezers
- Cheetos (*Can you believe it?*)
- Edamame

- Rice cakes with peanut or almond butter

- GF Pizza Bagels: GF bagel topped with tomato sauce and mozzarella

- GF Pasta with butter and cheese

- Ants on a log, aka celery filled with peanut butter topped with raisins

- Quinoa mac and cheese (Add 2 tablespoons of milk and ½ cup grated cheddar to 2 cups cooked quinoa. Heat on the stovetop over medium heat for 5 minutes, and mix.)

- The almighty fruits and vegetables

This is also the time when your child gets invited to a crazy amount of parties. With the new "invite the whole class" rule so firmly in place, you're going to have to pick your battles. I would recommend going to the birthday parties only if a) the kid is a good friend; b) the parent is so awesome you can trust him/her to not poison your baby; or c) the goodie bags are said to be off the hook. Even then, send your child into the party prepared with his own dessert. You do not want your child crying in the bathroom because the rainbow layer cake looks so good it hurts her heart. That kind of temptation is incredibly difficult to overcome. Hell, I take a gluten-free cupcake to every kid's party I go to because *I* get all *verklempt* about cake. Don't let your child be the only one who isn't completely whacked out on sugar at the end of the day. That's just good parenting.

Another tip that is annoying but necessary: Always volunteer for the hospitality committee at your child's school, just to make sure the gluten-free contingency is covered. I hate committees too, but at least this one involves food.

Junior High & High School

Or as I like to call it, the "Age of the A-hole." At least I was when it came to listening to any damn thing my mom had to say. No matter if you have a celiac adolescent or a totally normal one, your kid is going to do things to make you crazy as soon as he steps into the hallowed halls of middle school.

Terror at the Arts & Crafts Table

Here's the other thing you have to worry about if you have a gluten-free kid: art supplies. Sadly, some of the kid friendly, eco-friendly fun times come with gluten. Luckily there are a lot of alternatives to the gluten-filled, so shop around and your child will not feel playtime deprived.

Not so into stressing out when your child is at school all day long? Provide your gluten-sensitive kiddo with disposable rubber gloves like they use at doctors' offices. Look for the smallest size, and make sure he or she's packing.

Play-Doh—The original brand as well as homemade contains gluten. And don't forget how much kids love to eat that stuff. Stay away, and find the gluten-free version.

Modeling Clay—Not all modeling clay contains gluten, but some do. Always check the label.

Papier-Mâché—The homemade kind is all about the flour, what with its sticky gluten.

Finger Paints—Sadly, some big-name finger paints are made with wheat, which is "nontoxic" to most kids, but not your little gluten barfer. Once again, always check the label.

(See Resources, page 230: Gluten-Free Toys & Art Supplies for Kids.)

Expect serious rebellion right now, including when it comes time for your hormone-addled offspring to eat. Try to put yourself in his shoes when he's sharing a pizza after the swim meet and just wants to feel like a regular kid for once. This kind of willpower is near impossible, especially for someone who does not possess a fully developed brain. Glutening will happen. Just try to minimize the damage by keeping your own home gluten-free and keeping an eye on his friends, those jerks. Also jerks? The jerks' parents. Your plan of action is to kill them all with kindness—and information.

As a parent to a child with food issues, you have to be way more up in his business than the average parent. You might as well get used to that idea and start introducing yourself to every kid's parents just in case your precious one winds up over at Johnny's house for dinner. Yes, this is just one more way you will be labeled "uncool" by your kids, but you're going to have to go for it. If this means making ALL CAPS announcements on the school message board, or standing up in front of the PTA, or just mentioning it every time you see a parent of a child who looks at your own with even a smidgen of interest—do it. Try really, really, really hard not to do it within earshot of your child. Hopefully at this point your kid is a soccer superstar or a mean fiddle player and isn't defined by her disease so this won't bug her. Still, it's cool to try to not make her feel like the odd woman out.

Other parents may find you annoying, kids will talk about you behind your back, and your own child may pretend not to know you. Yet this makes you not that much different from every single other parent of an adolescent. Embrace your inner busybody and get to know all of those people who interact with your child during the day. Just remember to be nice about it, and no one will be tempted to pelt your kid with chicken nuggets.

As only half of the equation, you still have to get your child on board. Kicking and screaming, maybe, but you've got to be a team when committing to the gluten-free life. At least until she runs away from home because no one understands her, least of all you. Try these tips to keep your gluten-free adolescent safe:

1. APPEAL TO HER VANITY

Remind your young gluten intolerant of all the weird skin issues that can happen when she consumes gluten, and don't gloss over the farting either. This is especially helpful on prom night when you're trying to keep beer out of her sensitive stomach. Do NOT use this on a twelve-year-old boy, however, because it will send him to the vending machine as fast as you can say "explosive diarrhea."

2. CULTIVATE A PERSONA

Remember when that first kid got braces in junior high? Before the sheen wore off the metal, everyone in homeroom wanted braces too. Teach your child to say things like "Yeah, I'll probably die young" and "I won't let this disease define me" to pick up chicks/dudes[*]. Note: Lines must be delivered with the proper emo face. From now on everyone around the table will involuntarily produce the sympathy frown when your child passes up the pizza and chews forlornly on a carrot stick. And that, kids, is how you become popular. (*Editor's note: Yeah, in the Drama Club, maybe.*)

3. BECOME AN ACTIVIST

Sure, preaching the gluten-free gospel can put some people off, but if your child happens to be one of those peppy cheerleader types who is all up in the awareness, she's more likely to stick to the diet. Whether she starts a blog, attends Celiac Disease Foundation conferences, or starts petitions for gluten-free school lunches, it will help her feel some control over her lot as well as encourage her to stay the straight and narrow course. You know, kind of like those Up with People kids. They turned out OK, right?

That, my friends, is how you keep your kids healthy and safe when the gluten attacks. What about the college years, you ask? Send money, gluten-free snacks, and pray every single night that your college student does not forget every bit of her home training the minute she moves into the dorms. Your work here is done. Now go enjoy that panini.

Oh, No! My Kitchen Has Gluten

Whether you're the gluten intolerant or your child is, if you have even one person in your house who is consuming gluten, you've got to keep their dishes

---

[*] Please rest assured this is NOT true and is simply a romantic device for your child. Yes, I realize that sounds bad too.

and their delicious food away from the others. My kids have cereal bowls that I never touch, and if they toast a bagel, they have to use a tray that my own gluten-free biz never comes near. Some days I think it would be easier to simply ban all gluten from the house, and then I realize how much more work would be involved in preparing school lunches without gluten, and I decide that preparing my own lunches is enough work. Making sure the kids are all gluten-free might just drive me nuts. Also, perfect ~~excuse~~ reason to transfer that responsibility—permanently—over to their father. *Amiright?*

But you're here because your kids can't eat gluten, and you will be preparing special lunches. The good news is your kid won't be the only one with an issue. You can't throw a Thomas Train into a playgroup without finding at least one kid who can't ingest a major food group. You are not alone, and I've totally got your back, as well as some recipes that will knock your kiddie socks off.

Although it's true that cooking with more complex gluten-free grains will be much healthier for your little ones, in the beginning I would recommend going for the path of least resistance. Which is why my kid-friendly recipes are all about making kids happy, even without that stupid gluten. Once you've conquered the all-purpose gluten-free flour, mix it up with a millet or a sorghum blend. Or teach your kid to do that, which would be way more awesome.

Recipes

Here are some recipes my kids chow down on like they're celiacs (which they're not, *thank god*):

Zucchini Muffins

My kids eat these like they're candy. It's one of those sneaky ways to get vegetables into their diet and also keep it g-free. It's the perfect kid recipe if you're all about depriving your children without their even knowing. Which we all are, right?

Prep time: 20 minutes **Cook time:** 30 minutes
Makes: 20 muffins

INGREDIENTS

1 ⅓ cup sugar
2 eggs, beaten
2 teaspoons vanilla extract
4 cups grated fresh zucchini
⅓ cup melted unsalted butter
2 teaspoons baking soda
Pinch of salt
3 cups gluten-free all-purpose flour
1 teaspoon xanthan gum
½ teaspoon nutmeg
2 teaspoons cinnamon

1. Preheat the oven to 350°F. Lightly grease the wells of a 12-well muffin tin.

2. In a large bowl, combine the sugar, eggs, and vanilla. Stir in the grated zucchini and then the melted butter. Sprinkle the baking soda and salt over the zucchini mixture, and mix.

3. In a separate bowl, combine the gluten-free flour, xanthan gum, nutmeg, and cinnamon. Stir these dry ingredients into the zucchini mixture.

4. Use a spoon to distribute the muffin batter evenly among the cups, filling the cups completely.

5. Bake on the middle rack until the muffins are golden brown and the tops of the muffins bounce back when you press on them, 25 to 30 minutes, or until a toothpick inserted in the center of a muffin comes out clean.

6. Set the tin on a wire rack to cool for 5 minutes. Remove the muffins from the tin and let cool another 20 minutes.

. . . .

Avocado Fries

My kid loves "green French fries," which come from a bag. So I naturally thought making my own gf green fries would be a winner. He eats something green, and I'm totally stoked.

What I didn't realize was that these (even vegan!) avocado fries are totally adult fare. Sure, your kids will eat them. But really, they're for you. As witnessed by my hoovering ten of them when I was trying to convince my son they were better than store bought. We thumb wrestled for the last avocado fry. True story.

Prep time: 10 minutes **Cook time:** 7 minutes
Makes: 16 fries

INGREDIENTS

Oil for frying
1 cup Better Batter gluten-free seasoned flour mix
2 ripe avocados, flesh scooped from the skin, pitted, and sliced into strips

1. Preheat the oil in deep-fat fryer until it reaches medium-high setting (alternatively, heat enough oil in a deep saucepan to submerge the avocado strips completely).

2. In a medium bowl, whisk the gluten-free flour mix and ½ cup water together until smooth.

3. Place the avocado slices in the batter to coat. Allow them to sit in the batter for 5 minutes.

4. Fry the avocado slices, turning every few minutes, for 7 minutes, or until the coating is golden brown in color. Drain on paper towel–lined plate to remove excess oil, and serve.

. . . .

Gluten-Free Chocolate Chip
Ice Cream Sandwich

This is a rad parenting move. If you make homemade gluten-free chocolate chip ice cream sandwiches for your kid and her friends, no one is going to complain about the lack of gluten. Plus, you'll pretty much be the coolest mom in the entire neighborhood.

You can also make these chocolate chip cookies solo, but why would you do that when you can fill them with delicious ice cream?

Prep time: 15 minutes + 90 minutes rest time   **Cook time:** 13 minutes
Makes: 15 ice cream sandwiches

INGREDIENTS

3½ cups all-purpose gluten-free flour

½ teaspoon xanthan gum

1½ teaspoons baking soda

¾ teaspoon salt

2 sticks unsalted butter

¼ cup turbinado sugar

¼ cup granulated sugar

1¾ cups brown sugar

2 eggs, at room temperature

2 teaspoons vanilla extract

½ pound dark chocolate, roughly chopped

1 quart vanilla ice cream

2 cups gluten-free chocolate chips

1. Preheat the oven to 375°F.

2. In a large bowl, sift together the flour, xanthan gum, baking soda, and salt. Set aside.

3. Using a hand mixer, cream the butter and the sugars until light and fluffy. Add the eggs, one at a time, beating well to incorporate after each addition. Add the vanilla, then scrape down the sides of the bowl.

4. Add the flour mixture and mix to combine. Fold in the chopped chocolate with a spatula.

5. Cover the bowl and refrigerate the dough for 30 minutes.

6. Roll the chilled dough into balls 2 inches in diameter and place them on a cookie sheet, ½ inch apart. Bake for 13 minutes.

7. Remove the cookies from the oven and allow to cool for at least 30 minutes.

8. About 10 minutes before the cookies have cooled completely, remove the ice cream from the freezer to soften it. Place the gluten-free chocolate chips on a flat tray.

9. Take 2 cookies of equal size and place one upside down on a flat surface. Using an ice cream scoop, place two and a half scoops of vanilla ice cream on the cookie. Place the other cookie on top and squeeze together to distribute the ice cream evenly between the cookies. Use a table knife to smooth the edges, if needed.

10. Roll the edges of the ice cream sandwiches in the chocolate chips until coated, then immediately wrap the ice cream sandwiches in plastic wrap and transfer to the freezer. Freeze for 15 to 20 minutes before serving.

· ·

Butternut Squash Mac & Cheese

My friend Noelle showed up to a dinner party with this dish and I was all, "Why you want to ruin mac and cheese like that?" Then I saw my picky eater chow down, and I demanded that Noelle send me the recipe, stat.

If your kids are like every kid since the dawn of man (including mine), they hate vegetables and love Wonder Bread. But now they're g-free, and you're super worried about their nutrients. Never fear! Sneaky butternut squash mac and cheese is here. Smile with satisfaction as they totally eat that winter squash and think they're getting away with something.

Recipe note: You can also use all-purpose gluten-free flour in this recipe. I happen to like the way millet flour works in a roux, so that's my go-to.

Prep time: 20 minutes **Cook time:** 1 hour and 15 minutes
Makes: 16 servings

INGREDIENTS

For the Squash:
1 butternut squash, peeled, seeded, and chopped into 1-inch cubes
1 tablespoon olive oil
1 teaspoon salt
1 teaspoon pepper
½ teaspoon nutmeg

For the Pasta:
1 pound gluten-free elbow macaroni
¼ cup unsalted butter
½ cup millet flour
4 cups milk
Salt
Freshly ground black pepper
1 teaspoon nutmeg
1 tablespoon dry mustard
4 cups grated sharp cheddar
1¾ cups vegetable stock

1. Make the squash: Preheat the oven to 400°F.

2. Place the squash in a large bowl and coat the pieces with the olive oil, salt, pepper, and nutmeg. Transfer the squash to a sheet pan and roast for 45 minutes, or until fork tender. Remove the squash from the oven and turn the oven up to broil. Set the squash aside to cool.

3. Make the pasta: Bring a large pot of salted water to a boil. Add the gluten-free macaroni and cook until al dente, 3 to 4 minutes less than directed on the package. Drain and rinse the macaroni.

4. While the macaroni is cooking, melt the butter in a Dutch oven or large saucepan over medium heat. Whisk in the flour, stirring constantly, until it lightens and thickens into a paste.

5. Remove the mixture from the heat and add milk, then return to the heat and whisk until the roux thickens. Reduce the heat so the mixture is just simmering, and cook, stirring frequently, until the roux thickens further, 8 to 10 minutes.

6. Transfer the squash to the bowl of a food processor or blender and purée. Set aside.

7. Season the roux with salt, pepper, nutmeg, and dry mustard. Add 3 cups of the cheddar and the vegetable stock to the roux, and mix to combine. Remove from heat, and add the puréed squash.

8. Toss the squash mixture with the pasta, then transfer the mixture to a large casserole dish. Top the mixture evenly with the remaining cheddar.

9. Place the casserole under the broiler for 15 to 20 minutes, until bubbly and brown on top. Turn the oven down to 350°F and cook for 15 minutes more. Allow to cool before serving.

· ·

Aunt Loretta's Deconstructed Lasagna

Aunt Loretta comes through yet again with a totally delicious way to make kids feel like the norms, in an incredibly easy move that does not require you to have the counter space to lay out long noodles. Also, my kids really hate lasagna noodles for some reason. Weird.

Prep time: 15 minutes **Cook time:** 45 minutes
Makes: 12 servings

INGREDIENTS

½ pound ground beef
1 teaspoon salt
Dash of freshly ground black pepper
1 teaspoon sugar
2 (8-ounce) cans tomato sauce
1 (12-ounce) package gluten-free pasta
1 cup sour cream
3 ounces cream cheese, softened
1 teaspoon oregano
½ cup shredded mozzarella

1. Preheat the oven to 350°F. Grease a 12-by-8-inch casserole dish.

2. In a large skillet over medium heat, brown the ground beef.

3. Drain the fat from the skillet. Add salt, pepper, sugar, and tomato sauce to the ground beef and simmer over medium heat for 15 minutes.

4. Cook the gluten-free pasta according to the package directions.

5. In a small bowl, combine the sour cream, cream cheese, and oregano and set aside.

6. Place half of the cooked gluten-free pasta on the bottom of the prepared pan. Cover with half of the sour cream mixture, then half of the meat sauce.

7. Repeat the layers, then top the last layer of meat sauce with mozzarella. Bake for 30 minutes.

Ice Cream Cone Cupcake

Another recipe to bust out at parties. There are some super-delish gluten-free ice cream cones, sprinkles, and cake mixes out there that make this recipe a snap. If you don't have a gluten-free cake mix handy, see my recipe for devil's food cake, and whip up a buttercream frosting that is naturally gluten-free. Add gluten-free food coloring and/or sprinkles and sit back and wait for the accolades.

VEGAN ALERT: You can easily make these cupcakes vegan because most gluten-free ice cream cones and cake mixes are vegan to begin with. In the icing, substitute vegetable shortening for butter, using 2 tablespoons less, and substitute water for milk, and you're all set.

Prep time: 15 minutes **Cook time:** 45 minutes
Makes: 12 cupcakes

INGREDIENTS

12 gluten-free flat-bottomed ice cream cones
1 box gluten-free cake mix, as directed, or 1 recipe Jack's Devil's Food Cake (see page 93)

For the Buttercream Icing:
1 cup unsalted butter, at room temperature
4 cups confectioners' sugar
½ cup milk
½ teaspoon almond extract
¼ teaspoon salt
3 drops food coloring of your choice, if desired

4 tablespoons gluten-free sprinkles

1. Preheat the oven to 350°F.

2. Set the gluten-free ice cream cones in the wells of a muffin tin.

3. Prepare the cake batter as directed on the package.

4. Fill each cone almost to the top with the cake batter. Bake for 25 minutes, or until a toothpick inserted in the center of a cupcake comes out clean. Set aside to cool for at least half an hour.

5. Make the buttercream icing: Using a hand mixer, combine all the ingredients except the food coloring and beat until smooth. Add food coloring, if desired, a few drops at a time, until you reach the color you want.

6. Use generous amounts of icing on each cupcake, to make them look like ice cream cones. Top the cupcakes with sprinkles.

Chapter Seven

TRAVELING WHILE

Sprueing :

PARIS DOESN'T HAVE TO SUCK, BUT IT MIGHT

Now that you have mastered the gluten-free cooking, discovered your local gluten-free hot spots, and are feeling totally confident about this whole new way of life, it's time to take a vacation! Although you can't take a vacation *from your problems*, you can work hard to not create more while you're out of your element. I'm talking about gluten problems here and how to solve them when you don't have your own kitchen handy. That's why you're here, right?

The great news is, any domestic travel you take on in the U.S. of A. can be solved by marching into two places upon your arrival in a strange locale: Whole Foods (or any natural food store) and a taco stand. Please note: This does not apply to camping. If you're seriously willing to go camping, you pack your own food. I, however, have decided my celiac disease is the perfect excuse to never have to sleep outdoors ever again. Ever.

Once you find yourself in a new city, head straight to the store and load up on g-free emergency food in case you wind up at the local pizzeria starving and angry. Also, refer to Chapter 4 to make sure you *don't* actually wind up at the local pizzeria, and instead find yourself happily munching away at the taco stand. If you're visiting friends and family, you can ask them to grab a few things or ship them a box of nonperishable foodstuffs beforehand.

And if you happen to be visiting super-amazing awesome friends and family, those people will look upon your stay as an adventure and will have already stocked up on the best gluten-free pasta in town. Also, bring those people presents because they rock.

"But April," you say, "I like to travel to places off the beaten path. I doubt there's a Whole Foods where I venture." Guess what, America? I just read about a contest where you could enter to win a $500 gluten-free shopping spree from Walmart. Which means they've got to have at least $500 worth of products, or else you get a consolation prize of Fritos and a "Born 2 Sk8" tank top. I kid. I'm sure Walmart is cashing in on this huge trend, because they know how to make the big bucks. Which means you and I have no more excuses to not visit our rural relatives. If Walmart can offer you gluten-free food, and Walmart covers the U.S. like a blanket made in China, you will not starve when you're traveling around this particular country.

Don't forget—even if you have only a backpack and a small amount of change (and if you do, ummm, what year do you think this is?), you can stop at a farm stand for naturally gluten-free produce. Because another thing that has changed dramatically with America's food supply in the past decade is the hipsterization of the farmers' market. Those things are everywhere, even in the small town I used to live in, which totally didn't need one because everyone had their own damn farm.

With so many gluten-free options in grocery stores, chain restaurants, and farm stands, you can book your tickets to Anywhere, U.S.A. Honestly, if you haven't noticed gluten-free menus, cookies, stores, and random gluten-free Lady Gagas popping up everywhere in our country, you're not paying attention. We're good here in the United States, and I hear Canada is pretty rad in the gluten-free department as well. Go forth into the wilds of North America and vacation.

I, however, thought it might be good to push the old gluten-free envelope. Not unlike the Republicans in the U.S. Congress, I came to the realization that the French could potentially present a problem. Although the Italians are all over gluten-free pasta and bread, the whole UK area practically invented sprue, and you can live on amazing seafood and rice if you head to the Far East, France is filled with delicious gluten plus attitude. Which means I absolutely had to get there, and fast. Masochist much?

Paris, It's ON

"Perhaps going to Paris isn't a great idea right now," my husband said right before I kicked him in the shins. Or thought about kicking him in the shins. Or really wanted to kick him in the shins because he was right. I'd just had my endoscopy checkup (wheeeee!), and the news was not awesome. As in "Hey, are you sure you aren't still eating gluten like a beast?" I was getting sick a few times a week, and incredibly busy uncovering sneaky gluten and its sneaky ways (see Chapter 2). Also, I had just had a wicked bout with the stomach flu because I'm lucky like that. Yet off I went into the wilds of baguettes, croissants, and waiters who already thought I was a horrible American, just to see if I could. At least that two-week stomach flu meant I was looking fabulous. *Watch out, Paris*, I said to myself, *because I'm about to be in you.*

But first, I had to get there.

Gluten-Free Airline Travel

The fact is every time you get on an airplane you'd better pack snacks—whether you're gluten-free or just like to eat food to live. Gone are the days with the waitresses in the sky who cater to your every whim. Hello, miniature snacks and pay-to-eat boxes of food that you, the gluten intolerant, cannot even eat. If you're taking a four-hour flight, this is no big deal. Try crossing the Earth, and it suddenly becomes a disaster of massive proportions. Why? Because you'll eat all of your gluten-free brownies on the first leg, and your string cheese will smell ripe by the time you're in your fourteenth hour of nonrefrigeration.

Contacting your airline before your trip is crucial if you're, say, in California and crossing like five or eight time zones in order to wind up in Paris. I was lucky that my airline of choice, Air Canada, provides a gluten-free meal when you travel internationally. Proof yet again that Canada has got it going on when it comes to the gluten-free. Then it occurred to me that if Travelocity had sent me in a different direction, I might have wound up totally screwed.

First, I made some calls. Although some people (ahem, Delta, ahem) don't want you to even talk to them, e-mail them, instant message them, text them, or, god forbid, send them a letter, other airlines were very forthcoming about their total lack of food options for the gluten-free. (In Delta's defense, they were kind of in a huge merger at the time, and now appear to be on the gf tip.) Here's what happened when I did some investigative reporting.

Gluten-Free Dinner in the Sky

I've told you how awesome Air Canada is with their gluten-free offerings. You do need to call every airline before you travel just to make sure the policy is still in place, so you can take full advantage of their special meals. Here's the word from other airlines about their in-flight gluten-free options (at the time of publication).

Alaska Airlines—Alaska Airlines will hook you up with a gluten-free picnic pack that currently includes hummus, gluten-free chips, almonds, fruit, olives, and fair-trade chocolate. That sounds delicious, doesn't it?

Virgin America—At the time of publishing, Virgin America was developing gluten-free options for domestic flights. This means as you read this, gluten-free is ON when you fly Virgin America. Whoo! So you can check out that cutie in seat 14F while snacking g-free.

Virgin Atlantic—Not surprisingly, the international arm of Virgin will have a full-on gluten-free meal available for anyone who calls within forty-eight hours of the flight. Instead of a complete makeover, the chefs replace gluten containing items in the usual meal with gluten-free options.

JetBlue—Snack yourself silly on JetBlue without worrying about the gluten. In addition to three free snack options that are gluten-free, you can purchase a gluten-free "Shape Up" snack box that is gluten-free, along with à la carte items.

Southwest Airlines—Known for peanuts, and that's it, so you can totally eat gluten-free on Southwest. Because peanuts are gluten-free. When I contacted their press office, they also sent me a flyer with a Jack and Coke option (to purchase). Which means Southwest is gluten-free and ready to party.

American Airlines—A little bit complicated, but if you sit back I can explain. If you're flying first class on American, you will get the gluten-free hookup in meal form. If you fly first class on flights for more than two hours, you will receive a complimentary meal. And if you ring them twenty-four hours in advance, you can even get a complimentary gluten-free meal (some of which sound quite lovely—sweet chili salmon, anyone?). Main-cabin domestic fliers need to bring their own gluten-free food. International is another story, where you can again request a gluten-free meal. Depending on the leg, if you're flying in the main cabin you will have a meal-for-purchase. However, if you're fancy and first class, it's on the house.

Lufthansa—You know the Germans are efficient, and when it comes to feeding their passengers they are even more so. On every flight that offers a meal, you can get a gluten-free version as well. Lufthansa sent me photos of omelets, polenta, and lots of fresh fruit. I have to say it even looked appetizing. So what flights offer meals? If you're traveling business class, any flight over two hours. If you're traveling economy, then your flight needs to be three and a half hours or longer.

Spirit Airlines—Bring your own food on Spirit Airlines because the snacks for purchase are chock full o' gluten, with the exception of the peanut M&Ms.

US Airways—US Airways did not have any idea, so the nice lady referred me to LSG Chefs, the airline's primary caterer. Although the US Airways rep did warn me that it was difficult to get a response from LSG, I was still surprised at the complete lack of concern. Perhaps they hate the gluten-free at LSG. I wouldn't know *because they never responded.*

Delta—If you're making a short domestic jump in the United States, Delta offers a few snacks that are gluten-free, like M&Ms and almonds. If you're lucky enough to be flying internationally, or on a flight that is longer than six hours, you can request a gluten-free meal by logging onto the "My Flights" section of Delta's website and requesting at least twenty-four hours in advance.

It might be enough to inspire a letter-writing campaign for the gluten-free cause. It might be, until you realize it's airline food. You are not going to be stoked even if it's gluten-free. Is it awesome to have the gluten-free option? Totally. Especially if you're traveling back from a country that could give two *les poops* about your gluten-free condition. But airline food is not the place to go to get a great gluten-free meal. You knew that already, right? Let's move on.

Arriving in Hostile Territory

The real problem in going to Paris gluten-free—when you're me—is the intimidation factor. From the waiter who took his smoke break *right next to my face*, to the fast-talking toddlers who totally know French, Paris makes me feel inferior. Sure, I'm of the Cajun type, so I should be able to claim some kind of grandfathering or something. (Note to France: You should totally do that thing that Israel does with its American Jews so all of us Frenchies can come live in your beautiful country and muck it up for a bit. *Non?*) Instead I wind up trying to fit in with my rudimentary French, and even consider lying to the handsome Frenchman who rents me my *appartement* and when asking about my French research says, "But surely you do not have the food allergy, *non?*" I just gave this man like a thousand bucks, and still I feel like I have to hide not only my Americanisms but also my gluten problem. Oddly, I admitted that I had celiac, but added, "I used to live in New York." You know, because everyone just adores New Yorkers! Which is when I realize this Paris trip is going to make me look like such an asshole.

Luckily my husband has a childhood friend who is full-on Parisian, and so we tapped her to give me lots of tips about eating in Paris. The most important tip? Don't go to Paris in July or August because so many people are on vacation. Sadly I discovered this after purchasing a nonrefundable round-trip ticket for August. You know who especially loves to go on vacation during July and August? Gluten-free bakers who have just opened a gluten-free bakery that looks like the most amazing store in all the world. I was the recipient of tons of tips on gluten-free bakeries and gluten-free–friendly restaurants because apparently Paris is getting with the gf program these days. Of course every single one of those amazing places was closed up when I arrived in town. Who can blame them? I was on vacation too. And so my awesome eating and working vacation was off to a whimper.

After convincing my temporary landlord that I was a cool New Yorker, and not at all weird because I had a disease, I stumbled around Montmartre looking for a café and quickly had my very first Parisian panic attack. Even though it was the wee hours of the morning in California, it was brunch time in Paris. Or whatever it is they do at brunch. Because all I could see for miles were coffee, cigarettes, and bread. I pulled up a seat at Café Le Saint Jean and instantly freaked out as I suddenly realized I had no idea what I was doing, even though I should have realized this years ago. A quick look around offers me no clue, as the Parisians are simply sipping their coffee and staring into the *rue* because *that's what French people do.*

I'm not sure when I noticed that I was not breathing at all, but my paralysis resulted in my first mistake when I ordered two cups of coffee. Jean-Pierre (as I call him) looks at me quizzically and holds up two fingers: "*Deux?* Or *un?*" I think briefly about pretending that I was ordering for two people, or maybe I had one of those "The Artist" dogs like everyone else in Paris who just happens to enjoy coffee, but ultimately decide to answer truthfully and panicky, "*Un! Un!*" Yeah, I'm doing great. Also, apparently I'm having coffee for breakfast. Or rather I had an espresso since I forgot the *au lait.* Oh. My. God. I suck at Paris.

Just as I've resigned myself to the fact that I will have to live on coffee and wine the entire time I'm in Paris—and also begin to consider taking up smoking again—I see that someone has sat down and is holding a menu. Damn it! How did I not look up how to ask for a menu in French? Also, what kind of café doesn't just bring you a menu? A French café, that's the kind. Of course the fantastic thing about Paris is that I can sit at a café staring into space for hours as I quietly freak out on the inside about starving to death in a major metropolis. No one cares! So that's what I do.

Right about now is when I should be pulling out my Triumph dining card that tells the French that I cannot eat gluten in their own words, without my horrible accent. But *non*, I decide ordering an *omelette avec jambon et fromage* should be fine, and why should I worry that young man while he's on his third smoke break? (*Jambon et fromage* are pretty much what I'll eat for the rest of the trip, by the way.) You know, most of the time ham and cheese do not contain gluten. Not this morning, however! That's right, I finally figure out how to order some breakfast and I get glutened. Le sigh.

I thought I was soooo clever. "Propose you take a gluten-free romp through Paris," I said. What a genius excuse for a Parisian vacation! "What could go wrong?" I asked. You should know that toilet paper in Paris is not at all soft, and bidets are not as plentiful as one might think.

By day two I still have not told anyone that I'm not French and cannot understand French, nor that I have celiac and cannot eat gluten. This way, I decide, I can feel totally like a norm walking around the streets of Paris. Although I do suspect a few people may have figured out the no-French thing. For example, the waiter at the café where I ordered l'eau ten different times before I finally yelled "water!" Listen up, guardians of the French language: You should not make something so *nécessaire* so difficult to pronounce. I speak *le* truth.

I can hear you saying, "Seriously. Pull out your Triumph dining card, already." I will get mine out of my bag as soon as I finish this cigarette. What? I'm just trying to fit in given as this is the most time I've ever spent at a café that did not have WiFi. Which may also be why everyone in France smokes—no WiFi at cafés. The real issue is this: I came to Paris and wanted to act like I was just a normal, if not exceptionally cool, gal traveling around Europe by herself. I was NOT stoked to cultivate the image of the American lady with food issues. That is not the ideal way to go on vacation, and plus, cigarettes are rumored to put celiac symptoms on hold. Never mind that whole cancer thing.

Alas, I had to stop pretending and start getting real about five minutes after my steak au poivre landed on my table covered in a thick light-colored gravy rather than the black peppercorn edging I was expecting. Here's another tip: You will make the Parisian waiter much angrier if you tell him you can't eat gluten *after* your food arrives. Which may result in you being the recipient of an incredibly tough piece of meat that was most likely washed off in the sink and thrown back on your plate, as well as the admonishment to "Just say it in English." So sorry about that mixup, Le Consulat in Montmartre! And fuck you.

Next stop, the crêperie! Don't scoff, as I learned right before I left that many crêpes in France are made with buckwheat. Holy gluten-free goodness!

Why yes, I could eat crêpes for every single meal, alternating the savory and the sweet. Yet I'm highly suspicious when I sneak peeks and smells of these delightful wonders. Thanks to my friend Wikipedia, I learn that *les galettes* are buckwheat; otherwise the crêpes are made with wheat—or *blé*. Tragically, the first five crêperies I go to all make the *blé* version. But since I have perfected my French phrasing, I continue to ask, *"Galette ou blé?"* everywhere I go— hungry or not. Oh, who am I kidding? *I'm starving.*

Here is your French crêpe tip that makes reading this entire chapter worth every second of your time: Buckwheat (gluten-free) crêpes are most likely to be found in the Montparnasse neighborhood of Paris. Big touristy areas? Not so much. You can tell just by looking if your crêpe is buckwheat or traditional wheat. Yellow and smooth? Don't make a move. Brown and spotted? You've got it! In spite of my mediocre rhyming skills, this crêpe information is the best information you'll ever have as a gluten-free traveler through France. Ever. Live it, love it, eat a *galette* or five.

I don't think I'm overstating when I use the term "tragically" when I say that tragically, I discovered the only buckwheat crêpe I had during my entire stay on the day before I left. Perhaps had I made that gluten-free find much earlier, I would have not reached the point where I stopped trying to please everyone with my impeccable restaurant ordering skills and instead cultivated a very French persona. Instead of saying *s'il vous plaît* and *merci*, I started to bark at waiters: *"Le beouf!"* and *"Non!"* It worked for me. Until I started feeling like a bad person and then wound up at a Chinese restaurant simply pointing to things that don't "look" like they had soy sauce all over them. Note to self: Must get much angrier before my next trip to France.

After that banner day where I went again to a recommended joint that was closed only on Thursdays (what the hell, Paris?), I hobbled into the café atop my Metro stop (another tip: Don't wear heels for hours of walking and sightseeing) hungry, tired, and unwilling to fight with yet another waiter about water. I order *de vin rouge* and—finally—pull out my Triumph dining card. Also, I straight up ask if they can't just bring me steak frites. It was my best meal in Paris.

Perhaps you're thinking that if one just used a Triumph Dining Card throughout Europe, one would be fine. Here's why you're wrong. Cocky with my successful meal, the next day I set out to buy some lunch to take back to my apartment. I'd seen all those rotisserie chickens spinning around and decided this was a gluten-free no-brainer. I stopped in the very first lovely looking *boucherie* and said (quite clearly, I believe) that I would like a chicken, please. Yes, totally in French! *I swear.* The *madame* of the joint then threw me for a loop when she asked what size. I pointed and smiled, and hoped I was getting a good-size chicken because what do I know from kilograms? That lady, who clearly had some unresolved anger issues, proceeded to grab these battered and fried potato lumps and she throws them in a takeaway box along with the *poulet.* I could tell this was going to go badly so I said, "*Non!*" (Which I've become very, very, good at, by the way.) She turned and looked at me like I was some kind of ugly American who had no idea that the rules of chicken include battered and fried potato lumps. Which, OK, *maybe I was.* Panicked and determined to get a delicious chicken, I then did what any gluten-free hungry person should do and fumbled in my purse for my dining card to explain why I could not partake of those delicious lumps of gluten. Madame took one look at that card and threw me out of her store. Which may be the first time I've been tossed for gluten-related reasons. At least that I know of. You just *know* that was the best rotisserie chicken in all of Paris.

Paris is an amazing city that everyone should visit at least once in his/her lifetime. The art, the culture, the food, and the romance of every single street corner you wander by—it's beautiful. But at this point, I was so fucking done and ready for my husband to arrive. Yes, I'm a feminist and big believer in independent travel for the ladies, but by then I could not wait for a man to join me for the weekend. Two reasons—one, he wouldn't let me get away with this "Well, it *looks* gluten-free" bullshit, and two, the man can *parle français.* Which simply reminded me of something I probably should have been thinking all along: Always take care of yourself as well as the person who loves you most would. I needed to start following my own advice and standing up for my gluten-free meals with or without that little card. Certainly the admission that perhaps I was lost without a man was a wakeup call to this independent lady. Until he arrived.

Lest you think my husband is a clueless gluten lover, I'd like to point out he had a thirty-six-hour journey due to massive screwups by the airline and only four hours of sleep during that same time, when he went on a croissant tear then wanted to make out in the street "because we're in Paris!" And then finally, borrow my toothbrush because his luggage was somewhere in the Frankfurt area. None of which was quite so maddening as when we sat down to a meal and he dug in to the baguette saying, "Oh my god, I could eat this for my whole meal, that's how good it is." So maybe only travel internationally with someone who is also gluten-free is all I'm saying.

The rest of my gluten-free Parisian travels went like this: I was pleasantly surprised by two restaurants that totally knew what gluten was. Two! I was lucky enough to meet a college friend at another amazoids restaurant where I ordered something that I assumed was gluten-free, then she spoke with the waiter until it was discovered that no, totally gluten up in there. (New tip: Maybe find a fluent French speaker to travel with while in France.) Finally I resigned myself to the fact that my gluten-free crackers purchased at the Naturalia food market, prosciutto, cheese, and gelato were basically the best ways to get through a Parisian vacation. That, my friends, is not bad. Not bad at all.

Right about now I can hear people saying, "Yo, April. You rented an apartment. Why weren't you cooking up freshness from the local farmers' market?" First of all, I don't know why you think you should sound so street when you're talking about cooking food from the farmers' market, and second, because there is shit to do in Paris. In spite of looking up every single farmers' market in the region, I wound up cruising the Seine, wandering through museums, and hanging out in the Latin Quarter as well as my own neighborhood of Montmartre. Although my apartment was awesome, I wasn't about to spend a good three or four hours shopping, cooking, and just hanging out inside. It was Paris, baby! And as I mentioned before, I was IN it.

No matter how many ridiculous ways I tried to speak French, got glutened, or simply tried to live on gelato and macaroons, the fact is now I feel confident in going back to Paris and kicking some gluten-free butt. We all know that we learn most from our biggest mistakes, and mine was simply underestimating my own fear of asking for what I need and being intimidated by beautiful French people. That, and the wearing of the high heels while walking up and down mountains multiple times per day. Oh, and not checking the local vacation customs before I hauled myself across the Atlantic. Other than those pesky mistakes, I totally ruled Paris and I'd do it again.

Traveling WITH the Gluten Intolerant

Maybe you picked up this book because someone you love is gluten-free and you're trying to understand her challenges. This is your moment. Having to curb your own cravings so as to not offend a gluten-free travel buddy is also not fun. In fact, it can be SO not fun that you may engage in an argument on the Champs-Élysées that ends in "If you love that brioche so much, why don't you *marry* it?" As the gluten-free person in this equation, I beg you to be patient with your patient. She does not mean it when she says the next time she takes a trip it will be to a "far, far, away land" where no husbands are allowed. Honestly. Also, she thinks it's totally sexy when you stand up for her gluten-free self.

Which brings me to this sad fact for the travel partner of the gluten-free: You also may have to avoid making out with your travel partner after you just ate your fifteenth French pastry. Kind of makes you think about your priorities, doesn't it? So yeah, traveling while being gluten-free, or with someone who is gluten-free, is hard. But look at it this way: It's your excuse to eat ice cream every day on vacation! Alternatively you could use your vacation time every year to go somewhere exotic and lose tons of weight. Just kidding! Totally do the ice cream thing.

I hope you've learned how to navigate your gluten-free vacation thanks to my massive mistakes and occasional wins. Just in case you do find yourself going to the most bread-covered location in the world, here are some more tips that will keep you safe and sound.

Paris Tips

• Don't go in July or August.

• Don't download French/English translation apps on your iPhone then neglect to get an international plan.

• Watch out for motorcycles and/or rent one.

• Don't get drunk and lose your hotel key.

• Learn how to request the check in French if you don't have two extra hours to spare. It's this: "*L'addition, s'il vous plaît.*" Also helpful, learning how to say "I'm sorry." It's this: "*Je suis désolé.*"

• Don't try to cram in a million things leaving you with no time to sit, relax, and enjoy that gluten-free coffee, wine, or tequila shot. You're anxious enough, what with the gluten thing.

• Rent an apartment instead of staying in a hotel. You'll have your own kitchen so you can shop for food and make it for yourself. You know, if you're more resourceful than I am. Also, refrigerators are good about keeping your wine and chocolates nice and chilled.

• When you're on vacation, at least one day should be devoted to napping.

Let's Talk About Frites, Baby.

There are a few ways your beautiful French fries can turn into an evening on the pot. If you're in America, it's usually because everything else is being fried in that oil, including the beer-battered shrimp. While in France, that likelihood goes down along with every citizen's cholesterol. You may be OK enjoying the frites all over France, but you should still ask. Sometimes those delicious fries are made even fry-ier by taking a dip in flour before hitting the oil. This is rare (in Paris, not Texas), but it happens.

Gluten-Free in More Languages Than You Will Ever Need

Afrikaans – gluten vrye

Arabic – خالية من الغلوتين

Basque – zeliakoentzat

Chinese – 不含麸质

Czech – bez lepku

Dutch – glutenvrij

Esperanto – gluten libera

Filipino – gluten libreng

French – sans gluten

Gaelic – glútan saor in aisce

Haitian Creole – gluten gratis

Icelandic – glúten frítt

German – glutenvrei

Italian – senza glutine

Latin – glutine liberum

Portuguese – sem glúten

Russian – клейковины

Spanish – sin gluten

Swedish – glutenfri

Turkish – glutensiz

Chapter Eight

JETPACKS FOR

Celiacs

Two words: "fecal transplant."

I'll tell you all about *that* amazingness in a minute, but first let's talk about the fact that even though we say gluten-free crackers are just as good as the regulars, all we really want to do is get our hands on some Premium Saltines. I know I'm not alone here when I confess that after my celiac diagnosis, my fantasy life switched from romantic encounters in the South of France with a steamy stranger to romantic encounters in the South of France with a baguette. Of course I'm going to whip up an amazing gluten-free dinner that makes me totally forget I can't have that delicious toxin, but I'm only human. And every now and then this human really, really, really wants some mother-scratchin' gluten.

Luckily—I think—as our gluten-free population grows and grows, there are more companies trying to make it possible that we can eat gluten again. You've got scientists working overtime, whether it's creating a chemical to make gluten-free bread look like real bread (Dow) or using your DNA to sort out the malfunctioning microbes in your gut. Really, it's an exciting time to be a celiac. Or rather, it's a less painful time to be a celiac. Because honestly, who in her right mind is excited about having an autoimmune disease? Not this gal.

I was, however, totally excited to talk with Larry Smarr of the California Institute for Telecommunications and Information Technology, University of California, San Diego, about fecal transplants and poo tea. No, I'm not an eighth-grade boy, but I was suddenly fascinated, and admittedly totally disgusted, by what could happen when you add more poop into the celiac mix. Kind of like doubling down on your digestive situation. Smarr explained the fascinating world of making your autoimmune disease switch off through the magic of human waste. You're paying attention now, aren't you?

I believe it's important to understand—even more for those of you who do not suffer from some sort of gluten-related ailment—that those of us who have the yucks are not even blinking when someone says, "Hey, you want to eat gluten again? You totally can. First, drink some poop. Oh, you don't want to drink it? How about we put someone else's poop up your butt?" OK, perhaps we're blinking. Maybe even blinking furiously when I put it so colorfully, but wait, it's awesome.

Admittedly what I spoke about with Smarr is a long way from becoming a reality as a treatment for celiacs. But a girl can dream, and currently I'm dreaming about eating a cupcake after receiving a fecal transplant. What?

Here's the deal. A fecal transplant could kick that autoimmune response right out of your gut—with no special drugs that you would need to take every single day. This is about to get complicated, but if I can wrap my head around it—and I had an Olympic weight lifter as a high school science teacher—you can too.

Smarr, aka pretty much the smartest man I've ever spoken with, has late-onset Crohn's disease and a vision of the future of medicine. He came to my attention through an article in the *Atlantic* that highlighted his unorthodox but thoroughly scientific method of keeping himself healthy. Smarr meticulously monitors every single thing going on in his body at all times, using blood work, stool samples, studying his own DNA, as well as the microbes in his gut. It occurred to me that this man who was also diagnosed later in life with an autoimmune disease that affects the gut would have relevant information for those of us with similar issues. Prepare to have your mind blown, people.

An astrophysicist and computer scientist who directed the supercomputer center that brought the Web to America[7]—yes, you can thank him for LOL-Cats; why not?—Smarr has been tracking his health through the maps of his body created through his regular information gathering via the whole DNA mapping/stool samples/blood work business. With the advances made in technology, Smarr and others believe that we will all be able to benefit from data obtained through blood samples and genomic testing. In other words, our DNA and blood work can tell us what diseases may be coming our way, how to prevent them, and what kind of symptoms we need to combat versus what another celiac may be dealing with instead, and a heck of a lot more. As Smarr pointed out to me, every celiac is different and has different physical symptoms, yet we're all being treated the same way. Naturally this goes for other diseases as well. Although his Crohn's disease affects a specific part of his intestines, others are presenting differently and require different methods of treatment. Using this information, physicians can switch from the business of treating an ill person to prevention, keeping symptoms of a disease at bay, rather than treating the symptoms once they're full-blown and most likely, painful. It's science, ya'll. And it sounds super amazing.

"But, but, but . . . April," you say, "I already have the sprue! What about me?" Which is where the fecal transplant and the poo tea come in. The colon—your colon—contains most of the immune cells for the body. For the celiac, especially the celiac like myself who develops the gluten issue in my thirties, the problem may be that the gut bacteria has changed and triggered the disease. Although you could live with the genetic markers for celiac for many years, one blow to the gut through illness, antibiotic use, or god knows what, and you are no longer able to enjoy a croissant. Change the gut bacteria back to a "normal" existence, and then maybe you can stop the autoimmune response. As Smarr puts it, "Autoimmune is a very specific software disorder in your body." We need to call IT and fix it. Or as Smarr explains, we could potentially undo the "persistent, bad ecology" in our guts by introducing healthy microbes and letting the bugs "fight it out" through the magic of poo tea and fecal transplants. Which, although disgusting sounding, are actually much less shocking when you realize it's about changing the microbial ecosystem in your

---

7 Bowden, Mark, "The Measured Man," Atlantic, July 2012.

gut. OK, still a little bit disgusting, but let's break it down.

The real-life practice of using poo tea to treat an unhealthy animal goes something like this: You've got a sick horse with a messed-up microbial situation. Take the poo from a healthy horse, make it into tea, have the sick horse drink it so it may ingest the microbes it needs. OK, so poo tea *is* disgusting, but poo tea can translate into fecal transplants in humans, which is the back-door delivery system of these same healthy microbes. Are you getting excited now? You should be! Except for the fact that no one is actually doing this for celiac patients at the moment. A few Crohn's patients are at the forefront of this research, but we are years away from seeing trials on a widespread basis.

When I was feeling squeamish about the idea of an experimental fecal transplant, Smarr pointed out fecal transplants have already been used on people who have contracted the potentially deadly *C. difficile* bacterium—with a 90 percent success rate. If this bacteria, which also affects the gut, can be knocked out using a fecal transplant, why not my messed-up microbes as well? Now you want a fecal transplant too, don't you? Hey, it's better than drinking poo tea.

It's also worth noting that Smarr mentioned something the paleo diet people say consistently: We were not made to consume dairy and gluten, and the people who can do it well are actually the people who were able to evolve somewhat. But for many of us, it's damaging. The theory being, then, that this stuff really isn't good for anyone, but especially not those of us who are not evolved. Wait, were we just insulted?

This way of reversing your disease is a long way off. Although I'd actually prefer a more "natural" solution to this whole celiac thing—you know, more natural than not eating gluten ever again—there are other innovations in celiac treatment coming down the pike that involve the pharmaceutical industry. I think it's clear from my enthusiastic use of refined sugar in my recipes that I'm totally not an all-natural hippie type. Sure, I prefer organic food that doesn't have antibiotics and pesticides all up in it, and yoga is cool. But if I have a headache, Tylenol will be going in me. I am up-to-date on all of my vaccinations, but I also believe acupuncture needles can solve a world of problems. OK, if I still lived on a farm in Oklahoma I would be classified as a full-on alternative lifestyle gal. Since I live in California, I'm just considered middle of the road.

Which is why I totally signed up to be a guinea pig in a clinical trial for a medication that could help the celiac peoples. Oh, that's right. I'm contributing to medical science! You like me a lot more now, don't you?

Alba Therapeutics Larazotide Acetate

Perhaps you too have seen the print and Internet ads looking for volunteers with celiac for a clinical trial, with those cute pictures of cartoon wheat stalks with big round eyes. Maybe you thought you had better things to do with your time, even though the wheat wanted to be your new BFF. I apparently do not, and so I decided to go for it. Yep, I signed up for a clinical trial testing medication on celiacs, in spite of the screaming fear in my head. Which is probably the first sign that you're making a bad decision. A very, very, very big sign that people write entire books about, so you should really listen. However . . .

This was not my first rodeo. When I went to school in Austin, Texas, I needed so much more money for beer. Austin also happens to have a thriving medical test kitchen (or whatever it is they call it—research?) where you can sign up for experiments and get enough money for the weekend. I will never forget that pain medication study where my wisdom teeth were ripped from my head and I was given the placebo. Ahhh, memories. Knowing this celiac study couldn't possibly be any more painful than that one, I was only uncomfortable when I went in to meet with the people running the study and sprained my wrist signing all of those waivers. Just in case it is not clear that you're taking a risk, if you enter into a clinical trial, you have to agree that they will not be held responsible for babies with five heads coming out of you. I was totally cool with that. Because you know what was on my mind?

- Krispy Kreme
- Umami Burger
- Deep-dish pizza
- Croissants (hell, even a Croissan'Wich)
- Magnolia Bakery cupcakes

I'll be honest. I was not thinking of all the good I could do the celiac community by offering myself up as a guinea pig. I was just thinking, *If I don't get the placebo, I'm totally eating all of those things.*

I know this is the wrong way to approach, well, anything in life, but especially a study that is trying to understand the elusive "leaky gut" of a celiac patient on the gluten-free diet and help those of us who accidentally consume gluten (which is just about all of us). By bombing said gut with a round pastry of sugar-coated gluten, you kind of aren't playing fair. Which is why I waited until the last day of the study to do so. *Or so I say.* This is also why I make a horrible celiac. It's like I'm just waiting for the day for someone to say to me, "Here's a pile of gluten; have at it." And when I say "like," I mean it is exactly that. Therefore, joining a clinical trial for selfish reasons is something I'm all about. It turns out I did benefit personally from this whole thing, and so my selfish desires were satisfied. Just not in the way I thought it was going to go down—with a giant pizza going into my gullet.

Of course the medication on trial was not meant to allow celiacs to enjoy gluten again with abandon; the purpose was for those of us with pesky symptoms to have a shot at some relief. Relief I wasn't even aware I needed until I started keeping records of my daily "activities" and realized that I did get sick with celiac symptoms way more often than I thought. I simply hadn't been as aware because when you go from nine painful trips to the bathroom every single day down to one or two, it feels GREAT. Still, that's not really supposed to happen if you're following the gluten-free diet. Which I thought I was.

Remember all that talk about cross-contamination and sneaky sources of gluten? This is why it's no joke. If you regularly engage in unsafe eating at restaurants or in your home, you will continue to feel like ass. Even if you don't feel like ass, your body will ingest gluten, and your villi will be destroyed. This will lead you to much illness, and eventually you will feel like super-ass. Which is exactly where I was headed—Super-Assville, Population: Me. This revelation caused me to go over my lifestyle with a microscope and, hence, discover even more hidden sources of gluten that were so sneaky, I didn't even THINK about the possibility. (See: gloves, Chipotle; Tylenol, generic; skinny vanilla latte, Starbucks.)

Friends, I learned a lot by engaging in this clinical trial. One, gluten is an even sneakier bastard than I realized, and two, participating in something that can help all of us is rather satisfying, even if I initially went into it with visions of cupcakes dancing in my head. I kicked more gluten out of my kitchen since discovering these bits and pieces were adding up, yet I still insist on enjoying a meal out in unsafe territory. As someone who simply can't put my entire life on hold and stay inside my home 24/7, I'm going to come into contact with gluten. If I have a pill I can take that will lessen the negative effect of trace amounts of cross-contamination, then that's great for someone like me. My hope is that by the time this book is published the clinical trial is even closer to completion and we'll see this drug on the market very soon.

But wait, there's more!

Alvine: ALV003

There are multiple drugs being developed to help us gluten intolerants become tolerant, or at least to not be completely immobilized by a glutening. In addition to the trial I was involved in, another pharmaceutical company, Alvine, is developing a drug (and moving forward quite quickly) that will help break down gluten before your immune system even knows it's there. Alvine's ALV003 is currently in even more clinical trials and seemingly on a fast track. Although this sounds amazing, it's still the kind of drug that is used for accidental gluten consumption, not one on which you can go hog wild and back to your old gluten-eating ways. Still, awesome.

BioLineRX: BL-7010

Another drug in the research stage is BioLineRX's BL-7010. I spoke with Dr. Leah Klapper, the general manager of BioLineRX, and what makes this study interesting is that BioLineRX is not a pharmaceutical company per se, more of a drug development company that bridges the gap between academia and pharmaceutical companies while developing medications. Thus, they have more freedom to explore and experiment with innovative approaches before dealing with the expense of development and human clinical trials. Which is why this medication is unlike the others; it's even more sci-fi like. Or at least it is to me, the layperson who did not even consider medical school on account of the blood and the math.

The BL-7010 came from work by a scientist in Switzerland and a university in Canada, and instead of being a pill to take to break down gluten, it actually escorts the gliadin as a whole right out of your system, like a doorman at a *Real Housewives of New Jersey* fashion show. A nonabsorbable polymer that gloms on to the gliadin, which is attached to gluten, this pill removes the gliadin from your body without affecting the digestive tract and reduces the amount of gluten exposure to the celiac and gluten intolerant.

So far mice have been the only living beings tested with this drug designed to attach itself to the devil gluten, and these tests have shown the drug to be safe for consumption and helpful in removing gluten from the system. BioLineRX's BL-7010 has yet to be tested on humans, but the hope is it will lessen the immune response to gluten. Not a full-on "Huzzah! I can eat gluten again!" medication, but one that could potentially chill out your body's crazy reaction to gluten when you dine out and aren't sure what they're doing with the dessert plates back there.

ImmusanT: Nexvax2

Although all of these possibilities are certainly helpful to those of us who cannot tolerate wheat, rye, barley, and triticale, how great would it be if all of us could just eat with abandon? SO great. The treatment that I'm personally super-stoked about is that celiac vaccine that you hear about but just can't believe is real. Nexvax2 by ImmusanT is in early trials, and the goal is to allow celiacs to tolerate gluten again after you've received a series of vaccinations. Since I'm already on the allergy shot train for dust, mold, and a variety of other living things, I say add in this one and I'll enjoy the outdoors *and* a sandwich. The trials are under way, but it will be years before all of the research is completed. Stay tuned.

The good news is there are lots of people actively working to make sure the gluten-free can be gluten-full once again, or at least not as damaged by the accidental—and inevitable—consumption of small amounts of gluten. The bad news is everything is in clinical trial phases, or not even close to clinical trial phases, so it's going to be awhile. Oh, and the other good news is we still can be healthy if we just follow the gluten-free diet and eat deliciously (see Chapter 3). I know I totally just destroyed my rep as a gluten complainer by saying that, but it's kind of true. It's clear (I hope) that I'm no Pollyanna, but in some ways we are lucky that rather than going on meds for the rest of our life, we just eliminate one delicious item for optimum health. And that, my friends, is where my Puritan/Oklahoma/martyr genes make their annoying appearance. So sorry, but they were begging to be heard.

Introducing . . . the Crackpots!

Since all gluten intolerants are different, it's impossible to say which drug, or which cure, or which supplement will help you with your gluten problems. But I will say this: Some of these people have got to be freaking kidding me. Like this guy, for a really stunning example.

Gluten Sensitivity Formula by
The Wise Alternative

Here's where I resort to my twelve-year-old self and call this the *stupid* alternative. If you have a blog, or a Twitter description, or even a T-shirt that announces your gluten problem, you've probably gotten an email or blog comment from J&L Health about their magical gluten solution. Led by Dr. Jack Wise and a Dr. J. E. Block, these guys say they have the solution, if we just give them a lot of money. Send the cash, and amazingly we'll totally be able to eat gluten again after taking their Gluten Sensitivity "miracle drug." As Block explains in his YouTube video sensation in which he claims to have healed celiacs, "There was no grain in the Garden of Eden." OK, so a) this has to do with your drug *how*, exactly? And b) who uses the "Garden of Eden" as a scientific argument? If you are not suspicious of their Gluten Sensitivity Formula by now, read on.

Here's the deal with the so-called Wise Alternative. These two dudes say they conducted a trial of 150 patients with people with "gluten problems." Later, they claim to have completed a double-blind study with twenty-seven patients, and 100 percent of the patients improved clinically. They say people were able to consume gluten with no problems, even celiacs. So where are these people, and why are we not all cured?

Let's say you're still intrigued. Here's what The Wise Alternative is asking you to do. Simply hand over your credit card to buy some pills—preferably one to three bottles—at $149 a pop. Wait six months, then send a fecal sample (another $99) to *their own lab* to be tested to see if you still have celiac, which, as we know, is not exactly how one tests for celiac. Additionally, these are the same people who have testimonials about turmeric curing cancer. So . . . yeah.

Next!

Alorex Celiac Management

Less expensive but even more vague, you can buy Alorex caplets for only $14.95. What do you get for $15? It depends on who you ask. I first stumbled upon an ad for Alorex on a site called FoodAllergySymptomsx.com (now defunct) where the claim was pretty enticing. According to the ad, one could gain the ability to eat wheat, rye, and barley. Alorex supposedly reduces inflammation and restores intestines' ability to absorb nutrients. Then I went on over to ProgressiveHealth.com, and I discovered something different about Alorex. That particular site loves to talk about gluten intolerance and all the horrible things that happen to our bodies, but if you look closely, it appears that Alorex is simply a vitamin that would replace those nutrients you lose when you are gluten intolerant or celiac. Vitamins are good, and most people who have an adverse reaction to gluten need vitamins on a daily basis. These aren't even particularly expensive vitamins, but it feels a bit disingenuous to talk and talk about gluten, when the reality is you're selling a vitamin. Just like everyone else at your local GNC.

GlutenEase

A pill that claims to absorb gluten if you wind up with a hoagie in your face, GlutenEase is a supplement that also promises to help your gut. I know a few people who take GlutenEase and say it offers them relief. Since the makers of GlutenEase themselves say it's not for celiacs, I'm not going to bother. The amount of gluten these enzymes absorb is minimal, so it's really like putting something else in your body for a tiny amount of help. You can decide if it's worth it, but this celiac will skip it.

The bottom line here is this: If these supplements suddenly allowed the gluten intolerant to eat gluten, wouldn't this be bigger news? Like, heralded all over the Celiac Disease Foundation and beyond? Again, I don't want to slam any and all alternative treatments, but if someone is trying to make mad cash money off your disease—just assume they are not in it for your health.

Personally I can't wait until I can eat gluten again and am looking forward to any legitimate method that would allow me to do so at no risk to my health, naturally. Of course, now that everyone is on the wheat-hating bandwagon (see: gliadin = poison), just when my celiac is beaten into submission, wheat bread products will be illegal in California. I just know it.

A Prayer for the Gluten Intolerant

O Lord/Lordess/Higher Power Who Isn't Judgey,

I know you have great faith in me and that you have surely not given me more than I can handle. After all, you promised to do that, right? Which is why I pray to you for guidance and assistance on this long journey through life without delicious, delicious gluten. But first—a side note: Seriously? You *really* thought life without normal pizza was OK? That I somehow deserved this type of culinary deprivation? I know you are all knowing, but come on!

I'm sorry, O great one, I just get a little frustrated at times. No matter, I will never lose my faith because, after all, you made us this way and as those adorable yet ornery-looking babies on posters tell us: "You don't make no mistakes."

Anyhoo.

So, master of the universe, I have a few requests. As I carry this burden of gluten-free eating through the delicious aisles of bread and pastry, please do something about the following for those of us who sacrifice so much gluten:

- The hunger in the belly that cannot be satisfied with quinoa
- Sample ladies with cheese on crackers
- Visions of doughnuts as far as the eye can see (that might just be me; if so, never mind!)
- Memories of happier, dinner roll-filled times
- Artisanal bread crumbs
- Gluten-filled office parties
- France
- That fresh-baked bread smell

Since you are all-powerful, I know these requests from a humble servant—a servant who totally can't eat the best things you have to offer, BTW—are surely doable. Oh, and if I keep faithful, do good deeds, blah, blah, blah, I'm just assuming that once I find my way to the ever after, I WILL be able to go gluten again. Right? Right?!?!?!

Eternally yours,
Gluten-Free 4 Life (but Hopefully Not After Life)

Chapter Nine

WHAT'S NEW,

Gluten?

So, you guys. It's been about two years since I told you all about the evils of barley malt and warned you about those jerky relatives who won't believe you about the whole gluten thing. Two years! That means it's time for an update. Instead of writing a holiday card filled with my (and our) achievements and challenges, I thought it might be better to just add on a chapter once *GIMB* went paperback. Just seemed more efficient than gathering up everyone's addresses. Also, less creepy.

Let's talk about what's new! Well, a lot more people know what the heck gluten is, so that's new. And I got glutened about fifteen times between when this book first came out and now, so that happened, and it sucked. (I told you, I choose my restaurants by closing my eyes and pointing to Yelp, and you shouldn't be adventurous like me. I told you.) I also learned to take my own advice re: vitamins and eating well. Most of the time. And the saddest thing I learned was that although I CAN make gluten-free crêpes and chicken & waffles every day, I probably should not. Which is why you'll find some healthier recipes at the end of this chapter; we can only have gluten-free chicken-fried steak so many times before our arteries start hardening. (I believe that number is 212 times, just FYI.) I'm incorporating more vegetables and less sugar into my go-to meals, and I'm going to show you how you can do that too.

I know. I've changed.

A lot of other things have changed in the gluten-free world as well. It feels like I'm on a crazy gluten-free roller coaster. One minute I'm sitting in New York City eating gluten-free fancy pasta at an actual restaurant run by a celebrity chef, and the next minute I'm being told that my whole disease is just a cry for attention. It's crazy, sometimes amazing, and a lot of times frustrating.

Let's break this down, shall we? Here's the latest in the life of the gluten-free.

More Products, More Problems

It's been a while since I was a newbie, standing in front of the gluten-free flour aisle grabbing every slick bag like it was the best kind of street smack. Just like a junkie, I was so scared of running out of my favorite sorghum flour once I'd sorted out how to turn my blend into muffins; I was convinced that the new strain would be "low quality." One time I actually walked out of Whole Foods with every single packaged food with a gluten-free label. Luckily, at that time they only filled two bags and just cost me half my mortgage, instead of all. But if I were to pull that stunt today, I'd be homeless. But not hungry!

Gluten-free is where it's at, and we can see it in every pasta, cookie, and cracker aisle we stand in front of, jumping up and down with joy. General Mills has added more than six hundred new gluten-free products to its mix[1], and I'm happily testing a new gluten-free beer what feels like every month. Having given up drunken Chex Mix parties after my diagnosis, I'm thrilled to announce I'm back on that (now gluten-free) wagon.

New gluten-free bakeries are popping up in almost every major metropolis. And mail delivery of gluten-free goods is available in those areas that are not so lucky to have gluten-free cupcakes on demand. Speaking of cupcakes,

---

1 http://www.lakenewsonline.com/article/20140809/Lifestyle/140809583

it seems that super trend is on the wane and the naturally gluten-free macarons are the "it" dessert of the day. There is even a gluten-free Girl Scout cookie. Or so I hear. My local troop did not get the memo, which is why I shun them as they hock their cookie wares outside of Ralphs once a year no matter how cute their little outfits are. Get it together, SU 505.

There are so many fantastic gluten-free expos popping up all over the country that it is impossible to keep track of the new gluten-free, celiac-friendly products on the market. According to Mintel, a consumer research firm, the gluten-free food industry grew by 44 percent between 2011 and 2013 and was expected to reach more than $7 billion in sales by the end of 2014.[2] It's actually getting difficult for me to walk into a restaurant where there ISN'T a gluten-free menu these days. (Before you throw this paperback across the room while screaming, "That doesn't mean it's safe!!!!" please see the "No Haters" section below for the cons part of this State of the Gluten-Free Nation address.)

On a recent flight on Virgin America, the Artisan Cheese Box included gluten-free crackers, just because. There was no "gluten-free" written on the box—they just had them. I have heard that you can walk into a medical marijuana store and buy gluten-free pot brownies, my friends. Which I would recommend, because if you're vaping, you're going to want to have something gluten-free and delicious close at hand.[*]

This is the great news. Of course, there is a dark side to all of the availability of gluten-free packaged foods, restaurant options, and, of course, weed. One, you're gonna get super fat. Two, at some point the trendies could leave us in the dust, and this has the potential to all go away, right when we find the perfect gluten-free Nilla Wafer. And three, gluten-free goods will put you in the poor house. Those of us who rely on gluten-free substitutes already know it's hella expensive, but did you realize that gluten-free foods cost 242 percent more than regular ol' foods?[3] That's why your kid won't be able to go to college. So enjoy those gluten-free chocolate chip cookies!

---

2 http://www.mintel.com/press-centre/food-and-drink/gluten-free-food-to-lose-weight

3 http://www.cbsnews.com/news/a-gluten-free-diet-how-much-will-it-cost/

* Do not take this woman's advice on ingesting or smoking substances that still remain illegal in most states. She is just a writer and not a good source of advice regarding impulse control.

Oh, right, and four, indulging in edibles filled with the ganja is not something everyone should consider, even if it is gluten-free. I just thought I'd put on my "mom" hat and tell you that. You've been warned. Also, with all of these amazing gluten-free narcotics available, we're never going to be able to avoid servers, chefs, and friends who are totally high and think they're giving us something gluten-free but they're too jacked up to notice all the soy sauce in the marinade. Seriously, did you know that 3 percent of people in the workforce are high?[4] That includes doctors and hospitality staff. It might include gluten-free nonfiction writers. But probably not.

But They Told Me It Was Gluten-Free!

And now for a word about safe labeling and total B.S. labeling. Before The Food Allergen Labeling and Consumer Protection Act was executed in 2013, and required for businesses by August 5, 2014, there was not much (if any) oversight on companies who made "gluten-free" claims on their products. But now it's the law, baby, so I guess companies can get big fines or something if they break it. I mean, really, if you're trying to make extra money by putting a gluten-free label on your bread when it's actually full wheat, I think you've got other problems than "fines." The Food Allergen Labeling and Consumer Protection Act ". . . defines 'gluten-free' as meaning that the food either is inherently gluten-free; or does not contain an ingredient that is: 1) a gluten-containing grain (e.g., spelt wheat); 2) derived from a gluten-containing grain that has not been processed to remove gluten (e.g., wheat flour); or 3) derived from a gluten-containing grain that has been processed to remove gluten (e.g., wheat starch), if the use of that ingredient results in the presence of 20 parts per million (ppm) or more gluten in the food. Also, any unavoidable presence of gluten in the food must be less than 20 ppm."[5]

---

4 "I Was So High," *This American Life*, NPR, May 2, 2014, http://www.thisamericanlife.org/radio-archives/episode/524/i-was-so-high

5 http://www.fda.gov/food/guidanceregulation/guidancedocumentsregulatoryinformation/allergens/ucm362880.htm

So while we can now rest easy knowing no one should be sneaking gluten into our gluten-free goods, those of you who feel the 20 ppm ruling is still not good enough will probably not be totally happy. Me? I'm happy because a load of experts got together to sort out the 20 ppm quantity (which is an absolutely miniscule amount of gluten—we're talking parts per million) and declared it safe for celiacs. As a celiac I'm going to buy into that. If you've ever had a bad reaction to something that has less than 20 ppm, or if you're just not down with ppm, then skip the packaged goods and stick to the naturally gluten-free items on the edges of your store. Either way, my gluten-free friends, we've made progress. Go forth and spend your paycheck on gluten-free items willy-nilly, knowing you will be safe.

Kale IS My Friend, and I Should Stop Trying to Hide Our Love

I'm going to admit something here that may put my artery-clogging street cred in question: I fucking love those vegetables. That spray mist that happens right after the thunderclap sound effect in the produce section, the bright and dark greens regal in their positions, the crunch of fresh celery straight from the bin . . . I could go on and on, but this is already getting weird.

Look, I'm not here to bum anyone out, least of all myself, but the fact is eating loads of vegetables, fruits, grass-fed meats (if you're not a vegan/vegetarian), vitamin-filled grains without gluten, and lots of water is the best way to be gluten-free. I know. I'm sorry. As you've seen by the whole rest of this book, I'm very in tune with those feelings of deprivation the recently gluten-free possess. And I fought back those feelings with gluten-free fried foods. If you're still in that gluten-free glutton phase, I'm not going to shame you. I will, instead, shame myself. If chowing down on loaded nachos every day was the best way to be gluten-free I'd be the flippin' Queen of Gluten-Free, but nachos should be a "sometimes" food. Or at least that's what I've been told. By my doctor. After I gained twenty pounds going gluten-free.

So here's the thing: You can eat well, deliciously, and with serious flavor by just focusing on naturally gluten-free foods. I'm not going to lie. There are weekends (like maybe right this second) when I snack on Fritos and that lovely Fritos Bean Dip that goes so nicely with the crunch of a chip, but for the most part, to be healthy, feel good, and not bloat up like a Macy's Thanksgiving Day Parade balloon, stick to the naturals. Luckily I'm providing all of these new recipes at the end of this chapter to help you with that journey. Of course, I include dessert. But at least two of those desserts include fruits and vegetables. Sure, one of the desserts is a gluten-free Ding Dong, but what do you expect from me? I am not a machine, you guys.

Gimme Drugs

Now, let's review vitamins and the like. I've already talked about the importance of taking gluten-free vitamins when you're gluten intolerant and celiac. Even if you're following the gluten-free diet, you're going to have accidents that could knock you back out, and you're generally in need of more support. I mean, I'm not trying to tell you that you're not healthy, but . . . OK, let's be honest: We're not the healthiest group at the farmers' market. The medically gluten-free have problems, and some of those problems come in the form of malnutrition and problems with vitamin and mineral absorption. Hopefully your doctor or a nutritionist already talked to you about this—and I know I did in the previous chapters—but if you're like me, you need to hear it again and again and again.

So here it is: Eat foods that are chock-full of the vitamins and minerals your body so desperately needs. My BFF, kale, is an excellent vegetable to fill some of your needs. You're also going to want some of those superfoods like blueberries and quinoa and avocado. Get those vitamin-packed foods right into your diet alongside a load of water to make that machine run smoothly. While it's best to add those foods to your diet—vitamins are not going to make you feel as good as eating vitamin-enriched foods will—if you're someone with an autoimmune disease or problems with digestion, you've also got to take your multivitamins. And also your calcium and your potassium and your B-vitamins and your omega-3s. And especially the one thing that can really make a difference in the way you feel day-to-day, but I often overlook: your probiotics. You, of all people, have to keep your gut healthy. I prefer the kind that stays in the refrigerator because it's got a lot of live cultures happening. Since I've been taking probiotics regularly, I've felt much better in the digestive department. When you travel, count those babies out and take them with you. You don't want to get sick when you're on vacation or away for work. You want to be at your best. Take those mother scratchin' vitamins, you guys. Do it.

Oh, right, and one more thing: exercise. I know, I can't believe I just said that either. I hate exercise. I've never experienced that runner's high or the rush of endorphins after a particularly exciting spin class (although, admittedly I've never gone to a spin class on account of the rumors I've heard about vagina pain). Exercise has always been a chore for me, even when I was playing sports. Today, however, I am admitting to you that I need to exercise, and I'm telling you that you do, too. Please don't pelt me with gluten-free rolls.

The thing about me, and a lot of you who suffer from an autoimmune disease, is that my joints get inflamed during times of glutening and stress. It's your basic arthritis situation, and it does not feel great. While I can rub menthol gels all over my body until the cows come home, that's not really a day-to-day option. Nor is popping ibuprofen, since that's hard on the ol' celiac stomach. The only way to help our bodies stay strong during this fight is to make them strong.

Personally, I'm never going to be a marathon runner no matter how many times I swear I'm signing up for one. You may love running and get that high (lucky dog), or you might find swimming to be your jam. Whatever your favorite form of exercise is, I suggest you do it regularly to keep that compromised body in the best shape you can. I hate to keep harping on this, but we are not 100 percent well. We need all the help we can get, and keeping everything else working and healthy will go a long way to our increasing quality of life and longevity.

After avoiding every possible gym and exercise trend, I've finally come around to yoga and Pilates; they are truly great ways to keep your joints loose, strong, and healthy. Do I love them? I could do without all the "om"ing, and the sweating, and the driving to the places to exercise. So that answer would be no. But I know my body needs it, and if I want to continue living my super-fun life, I've got to get it together. You do, too. I'm sorry. Now, let's talk about food again!

Eat three times a day, and not on the run. Make sure you use food as fuel for your beaten-down body so it runs when you need it to run. I know I sound like your mother, and I know you really just want to get to the Ding Dong recipe, but I can't emphasize enough the importance of good food going into your gluten-free body. If you're really struggling, I suggest you start a dream board and fill it with pictures of kale.

We Can Eat White Vinegar Now! Hooray?

I, probably like you, was told a load of B.S. when I went gluten-free (see "More Lies About Gluten" on page 47). A lot of those lies were started by wheat industry groupies, I'm pretty sure, but some were long-held beliefs that had not been thoroughly tested. Thank goodness for my favorite Italian ever, Dr. Alessio Fasano, who has been knocking down gluten myths left and right, most recently in his book *Gluten Freedom*. One of the more surprising finds by Dr. Fasano, as outlined in his book, is that we no longer have to be afraid of white vinegar. Hooray! Easter egg dyeing is back on the table. But more important, for the adults, is Dr. Fasano's statement that booze that has been distilled is A-OK for the celiac. Now do you see why he's my favorite Italian?

There has been so much chatter about vodka, bourbon, and various other spirits having gluten (again, see "More Lies About Gluten" on page 47), and the fact is the process that makes these grains, roots, and sometimes fruits and vegetables into a lovely liquid that will get you loaded is safe for the celiac. This, of course, does not include any flavored liquors that include barley malt. But if you're just looking for a martini, go crazy.

Or don't. Honestly, if you don't feel good after drinking Scotch or vodka, please don't drink it. I'm not talking about the "don't feel good after drinking five martinis" kind of not feeling good, but I'm sure that's good advice too. What I'm saying is that if you indulge in an Old Fashioned and you feel gluten bombed after, stay away from the Old Fashioned. While science (and a top researcher) is saying that spirits are safe for us, you know your body. I would never suggest "just trying" a food, drink, or otherwise if your past experience has been decidedly negative. That's just mean. What I am saying is this: If you've been frightened by the Internet, a real doctor without the last name "Google" has given you the all-clear.

Get ready for more good news, gluten-free types. Although this good news comes with a major caveat, it's still exciting to know that caramel color produced in the United States is gluten-free. According to Shelley Case, who is a licensed dietician on the medical advisory boards of the Celiac Disease Foundation, the Gluten Intolerance Group, and the Canadian Celiac Association, while companies can use barley malt in caramel color, manufacturers in the United States are opting for corn.[6] Even in Europe, where wheat starch is used, the process is such that caramel color produced overseas is also gluten-free for the celiac. Bring on those caramel lattes with whipped cream, barista! That caveat I mentioned? Case made this statement in 2014, and I have no idea what year you're in as you read these words. Manufacturing methods can, and do, change. Always check the label and/or call a company to make sure your caramel color is gluten-free and safe for you to guzzle.

We Can Make Sandwiches

Oh yes, that white vinegar thing? Enjoy a ham and cheese with mustard. While we've been avoiding mustards that are made with vinegar, those days are over! Unless that mustard has a (gluten-filled) beer ingredient, Dr. Fasano says white vinegar is safe for celiacs, and I will listen to that expert. Although, personally, I scarfed down a few mustard-covered gluten-free sandwiches

---

6 http://celiacdisease.about.com/od/celiacdiseasefaqs/f/Caramel_Coloring.htm

before I heard the word that I wouldn't get sick, and now I know why I was fine. I mean, what was I supposed to do? Substitute mayonnaise? I'm not an animal.

No Haters (OK, 5 Bazillion Haters . . .)

And now for the bad news: As gluten-free grows in popularity, there are a lot of people who are seemingly really cheesed off about this state of affairs. Having grown up on a wheat farm, I can attest that it is not fellow wheat farmers' daughters who are leading this crusade, which basically comes down to this: You're gluten-free? I FUCKING HATE YOU.

This is happening, people. And you've probably been on the business end of this hate at one point in your gluten-free life. I'll tell you about my latest, which was actually pretty mild. I was enjoying a lovely gluten-free meal at a close friend's wedding when another guest (knowing that gluten was, indeed, my bitch) asked me if my meal was safe and delicious. So nice! What was not so nice was the lady sitting right next to me who turned to the person asking the question and said, "You don't really believe all of that gluten-free business, do you?" Since I was closest in location to the lady, I politely informed her, "Well, I do. I have celiac disease, and I'll get incredibly ill if I eat gluten." Instead of acknowledging that maybe there was someone with an informed opinion (in fact, the only person in the room to which this question even mattered), the old gal turned back to the original inquirer and said, "Well, do you?" I was all, "Bitch, give me your money." Except I wasn't, because I was at a wedding in the Hamptons and you know that would NOT go over well. Instead, I looked across at my friends who were surrounding me and rolled the hell out of my eyes.

This story is such a minor one in the field of famous talk show hosts shoving pie into the faces of the gluten-free (OMG, SO FUNNY. Not.) and children's television shows that advocate for the bullying of the gluten-free. While I don't like to deal with hostile and aggressive people who think the whole gluten-free thing is a personal affront, they will continue to exist long after they (hopefully) develop the debilitating symptoms of celiac disease or an autoimmune disorder. I kid. Sort of.

I don't want to compare us to the Kardashians, but let's go there just for a second. When the reality show *Keeping up with the Kardashians* first aired, people were intrigued by a mother who had been married to one of O. J. Simpson's lawyers for the murder trial of O. J.'s wife and her friend Ron Goldman. The lawyer who looked like he could not freaking believe it when Mr. Simpson was found "not guilty" by the jury. Who were these people? Was this a struggling mom just trying to move out of a very challenging situation after her horde of beautiful daughters (plus one so-so son and two more daughters with their stepfather) lost their father? We all wanted to know. Add in the Bruce Jenner factor to make it a modern-day Brady Bunch and wow, what is shaking up in Calabasas? Then, as soon as we realized this crew of brunette bombshells was going to saturate every inch of media, we turned on them. Yep, even Khloe. Stay with me.

You see, when there was a small, and very quiet, group of celiac sufferers and gluten-intolerant outliers, it was easy to pat them on their little gluten-free heads and move on. You felt sorry for this crew of people who would never have a baguette again, but mostly, you didn't think about them at all. Which is normal.

Then came the perfect storm of increased celiac diagnosis via awareness, the Paleo movement, and a dramatic increase in food allergy diagnoses. Now normal people can't get away from this crazy talk! They're pretty sure President Obama is coming for their gluten, and they are not happy. Naturally, they turn on those of us who are embracing (forced into embracing, but still embracing) the gluten-free life. Just as awareness of the Kardashians made people lash out against vocal fry, awareness of gluten made people lash out against those of us who say, "No, thanks" to French fries made in the same vat as that breaded chicken sandwich. They're done with us. All of us.

But just like the Kardashians (yes, I'm still beating the hell out of this analogy), you haters have got to understand: The gluten-free (and the Kardashians) don't give two shits about you. Not even one shit, honestly.

Maybe we should all let the gluten-eaters in our life know that no one is coming for their gluten. No one is going to make your gluten-y friends eat

gluten-free pizza when you dine out together. No one is going to ban croissants in the U.S.A. There are more gluten-eaters than there are gluten-pukers
and the dominant theme will always be the unlimited bread basket.

So tell the gluten-free haters to relax. They're fine. Us, however? We're
likely to poop our pants at any given moment. I'd say they have the upper
hand here.

The Big Gluten Picture

The gluten-free space is changing rapidly. While it seems to be changing to be
more accommodating to those of us who have to ditch the gluten, with that
comes some anxiety as well. Sure it's great that people know what gluten is,
but it's also a prime target for jokes made at our expense. It's also a way to be
singled out, bullied, and generally made to feel "less than." Forget all that. Go
get yourself some kale, crack open this book, find some ama-zoids recipes,
and go about the business of being you.

Recipes

FOR THE HEALTHY TYPES

· ·

Once you've had your fill of Beef Brisket Frito Chili Pie (page 87), you're going to want to fill up your gluten-free gullet with foods that are a bit more healthy. At the risk of alienating both the Paleo and the vegan crowds, I define "healthy" as "everything in moderation" and "eat your vegetables, like a lot."

Most of the recipes here are breakfast, lunch, and dinner options that I have added to my weekly rotation since I'm much more interested in filling up on vegetables and protein and not deep-fried gluten-free dough. The desserts, obviously, are not as healthy as the main course and breakfast dishes. Since I insist on still eating dessert, I included "healthier" options than say, my grandmother's Chess Pie (page 101). Bon appetit, GFers.

Baked & Stuffed Avocados

I love this for breakfast because it combines loads of my favorite things, and it's also filling! Plus I can be all, "I ate a fruit/vegetable for breakfast, everybody!" because I still don't understand what an avocado really is.

Prep time: 10 minutes **Cook time:** 15 minutes
Makes: 4 servings

INGREDIENTS

2 barely ripe avocados, pitted
4 eggs
Cayenne pepper
Sea salt
2 tablespoons grated Havarti cheese

1. Preheat the oven to 425°F.

2. Place each avocado half in a ramekin or small baking dish. Crack an egg into the hollow in each avocado half. Sprinkle with cayenne pepper and sea salt to taste and cover with the cheese.

3. Bake for 15 minutes, or until the egg is done. Remove from the ramekins and serve warm.

· ·

Almond Butter & Apple Sandwiches

I almost feel guilty calling this a recipe, because it's really just assembling sandwiches. But it makes for a delicious, healthy snack, so start apple cutting and almond butter spreading, you guys.

Prep time: 5 minutes
Makes: 4 servings

INGREDIENTS

2 firm, crisp apples (Gala, Honeycrisp, and Fuji are the best)
2 to 3 tablespoons almond butter
Honey

1. Lay the apples on their sides and cut them into slices approximately 1/3 inch thick, so that you get five or six slices from each apple. Cut out the centers to remove the seeds and the core.

2. Spread about 2 teaspoons almond butter atop one apple slice, and drizzle honey on top of the almond butter.

3. Top the coated apple slice with a plain apple slice to make a "sandwich." Repeat with the remaining slices.

4. Serve immediately or save for a perfect midday snack.

. . . .

Berry Refreshing Smoothie

Here's the reason I'm not so high on smoothies: I hate bananas, and I hate yogurt. You probably do not. But if you're like me, try this version for a mid-afternoon pick-me-up or a first-thing-in-the-morning pick-me-up. Also, bring a toothpick on account of the berry seeds that will be stuck in your teeth after drinking.

Prep time: 10 minutes
Makes: 4 servings

INGREDIENTS

2 cups raspberries
½ cup strawberries, hulled
1 cup orange juice
1 cup raspberry sorbet
Juice of 2 limes
2 cups ice, plus more if needed

1. In a blender or food processor, puree the raspberries and strawberries until smooth.

2. Add the remaining ingredients and pulse on "smoothie" setting (or "liquefy") until the mixture reaches the desired texture. Add more ice to thicken it, if desired.

3. Serve in a tall glass with a straw.

Coconut Rice with Toasted Almonds

This is a fab breakfast when you're feeling nostalgic about the days of oatmeal. You could also serve it as a side dish, but I'm a fan of a big bowl of steamy rice first thing in the a.m.

Prep time: 5 minutes **Cook time:** 20 minutes
Makes: 4 servings

INGREDIENTS

2 cups long-grain white rice
1 cup coconut milk
½ cup slivered almonds
Honey

1. In a medium saucepan over high heat, combine 2 cups water, the rice, and coconut milk and bring to a boil. Turn the heat down to low and cook for 15 to 20 minutes, or until the liquid is absorbed and the rice reaches the desired fluffiness.

2. While the rice is cooking, heat a skillet over high heat. Toast the almonds in the skillet for 2 to 3 minutes, stirring constantly, until lightly toasted.

3. Serve the rice in bowls sprinkled with the toasted almonds and drizzled with honey.

. . . .

Avocado & Kale Salad

One of my favorite restaurants in Los Angeles serves an avocado and kale salad that is tragically not safe for me to eat due to some flash-frying that goes on behind the scenes. I practiced re-creating its wonder using my husband as a taste tester, and this appears to be the winning combination.

If you're concerned about the ranch dressing component, use a light version, or maybe just don't think about it while enjoying this dish.

Prep time: 15 minutes **Cook time:** 5 minutes
Makes: 4 servings

INGREDIENTS

¼ cup vegetable oil
1 bunch kale, stems removed and leaves chopped
2 cups Brussels sprouts, trimmed and quartered
1 avocado, pitted, peeled, and cubed
2 tablespoons gluten-free ranch dressing
2 tablespoons roasted pepitas
Salt
Freshly ground black pepper

1. Heat the oil in a large, deep skillet over high heat until the oil begins to pop.

2. Working in batches and maintaining a safe distance from the hot oil, use a metal strainer with a long handle to drop the kale and Brussels sprouts into the oil, removing them after 30 to 45 seconds. Transfer the flash-fried vegetables to a paper towel–lined bowl after cooking. Continue with remaining vegetables.

3. Transfer the drained vegetables to a medium serving bowl. Add the avocado and ranch dressing and toss thoroughly.

4. Sprinkle the pepitas on top and season with salt and pepper to taste. Serve immediately.

Grilled Vegetable Salad

Grilling root vegetables is a great way to feel like you're eating something hearty while totally being ridiculously healthy. Hey, go crazy and mix it up with the seasons and swap out grilled spring veggies. I won't tell.

If you don't have an outdoor grill, you can also roast in the oven and/or break out that George Foreman that's been taking up space in the back of the bottom cabinet.

Prep time: 10 minutes **Cook time:** 15 minutes
Makes: 4 servings

INGREDIENTS

For the Grilled Vegetables:
2 cloves garlic, finely chopped
1 red onion, sliced in rounds
1 large sweet potato, peeled and sliced in rounds
1 acorn squash, peeled and diced
4 parsnips, quartered
1 beet, peeled and sliced in thin rounds
1 tablespoon vegetable oil plus more for the grill
Salt
Freshly ground black pepper
1 bunch mesclun greens

For the Dressing:
Juice of 1 lemon
1 tablespoon extra-virgin olive oil
Salt
Red pepper flakes

1. Make the vegetables: In a large bowl, combine the garlic, onion, sweet potato, acorn squash, parsnips, and beet. Toss with 1 tablespoon vegetable oil and salt and pepper to taste. Allow to marinate for 10 minutes.

2. While the vegetables are marinating, lightly grease the grill in two areas with a thin layer of vegetable oil. Allow the grill to heat on high for 5 minutes, then turn the heat to medium on one side.

3. Transfer the vegetables to the hot area of the grill and sear on both sides, 1 minute per side. Transfer the vegetables to the cooler area of the grill and cook for 10 to 15 minutes longer, or until tender. Remove the vegetables from the heat.

4. Make the dressing: In a lidded jar, combine the lemon juice, olive oil, and salt and red pepper flakes to taste. Shake well and dress the mesclun greens in a large salad bowl.

5. Make the salad: Add the roasted vegetables to the greens and toss. Serve while the vegetables are still warm.

- -

Fennel-Citrus Salad

Either you love the strong flavor of fennel or you don't. I absolutely adore fennel, so I like to keep this simple and clean so the distinct flavor is not overpowered. This is also one of those pretty salads you can bust out at a spring picnic and everyone will think you're super fancy.

Prep time: 10 minutes
Makes: 4 servings

INGREDIENTS

For the Salad:
1 bulb fennel, stems removed and sliced in thin strips lengthwise
1 bunch escarole

2 tangerines, peeled and segments separated
¼ cup toasted slivered almonds

For the Dressing:
½ cup red wine vinegar
½ cup extra-virgin olive oil
1 clove garlic, crushed
Salt
Freshly ground black pepper

1. Make the salad: In a medium bowl, toss the salad ingredients together.

2. Make the dressing: In a lidded jar, combine the vinegar, oil, garlic, and salt and pepper to taste. Shake well and taste for seasoning.

3. Dress the salad and serve immediately.

· ·

Roasted Gazpacho

Yes, I realize the point of making gazpacho is to avoid using your oven in the heat of summer, but the roasted flavor is what sets this recipe apart. The avocado makes it a bit more substantial, so you can act like you're having a real meal and not just soup.

Prep time: 15 minutes **Cook time:** 25 minutes
Makes: 6 servings

INGREDIENTS

2 pounds tomatoes, halved
1 red onion, thinly sliced
1 red pepper, cored and quartered
1 zucchini, halved

1 clove garlic, finely chopped

4 tablespoons olive oil

1/4 teaspoon sea salt

1/4 teaspoon freshly ground black pepper

1 avocado, pitted

1/4 teaspoon red pepper flakes

Tortilla chips, crushed, for serving

1. Preheat the oven to 450°F.

2. Place the tomatoes, onion, pepper, zucchini, and garlic on a baking sheet, evenly spaced to avoid crowding. Pour 1 tablespoon oil evenly over the vegetables. Lightly season the vegetables with the salt and pepper and roast for 25 minutes, stirring occasionally. Remove the roasted vegetables from the oven and allow them to cool.

3. In a blender or food processor, puree the roasted vegetables, half the avocado, the red pepper flakes, and the remaining 3 tablespoons oil to desired consistency, adding 1/2 cup water to achieve desired result (I recommend keeping it slightly chunky). Taste and adjust the seasoning. Chill in the refrigerator for at least 15 minutes or up to 1 hour.

4. Serve with crushed tortilla chips and the remaining avocado sliced on top.

. . . .

Broccoli Soup

This is one of those vegan soups that you can eat when you're feeling guilty about that gluten-free pizza binge you went on all week. Or maybe that's just me. If you want to stray from the vegan theme, you can use chicken stock and finish the soup with a sprinkling of Parmesan.

Prep time: 15 minutes **Cook time:** 40 minutes

Makes: 8 servings

INGREDIENTS

1 tablespoon olive oil
1 sweet onion, diced
1 large russet potato, peeled and diced
4 cups gluten-free vegetable stock
1 large or 2 small heads broccoli
½ teaspoon red pepper flakes
2 teaspoons sea salt
1 teaspoon freshly ground black pepper

1. Heat the oil in a Dutch oven over medium heat. Add the onion and cook until softened, about 10 minutes.

2. Add the potato and stock to the Dutch oven and turn the heat up to high, bringing the mixture to a boil. Reduce the heat to medium-low and cook for 10 minutes to soften the potato.

3. Prepare the broccoli by discarding the stalks and cutting the florets into small pieces.

4. Add the broccoli and red pepper flakes to the Dutch oven and cook for 15 minutes.

5. Remove the soup from the heat and add the salt and pepper. Allow to cool for 10 minutes before transferring to a food processor or blender and blending until smooth. Serve while warm.

. . . .

Radicchio, White Bean & Bacon Soup

I love white beans. I would eat them on almost anything, in anything, mashed into any shape. When you combine radicchio and bacon with white beans, well, it's just about the best soup you'll ever have. (Note: Go veggie by losing the bacon and using gluten-free vegetable stock instead of chicken.)

Prep time: 15 minutes **Cook time:** 35 minutes
Makes: 6 servings

INGREDIENTS

½ cup olive oil
½ sweet onion, diced
2 teaspoons chopped fresh thyme leaves
2 cloves garlic, finely chopped
½ cup dry white wine
1 teaspoon sea salt
1 teaspoon white pepper
1 medium head radicchio, roughly chopped
3 (15-ounce) cans white beans, drained
4 cups gluten-free chicken stock
4 strips bacon, cooked and crumbled

1. Heat the oil in a Dutch oven over medium heat. Add the onion, thyme, and garlic and cook for 5 to 7 minutes, until the garlic and onion are soft.

2. Add the wine, salt, and pepper and cook for 5 minutes.

3. Turn the heat down to low and add the radicchio. Cover and allow to steam for 5 minutes.

4. Turn the heat up to high and add the beans and stock. Bring to a boil, then reduce the heat to low and cook for 20 minutes or until the soup has reached the desired consistency. Add water and season with more salt if necessary.

5. Serve the soup in bowls topped with the bacon crumbles.

Grilled Shrimp Kabobs

Kabobs are the easiest thing ever. You put meat on a stick and put it on the grill. The one trick to avoid burning those kabob sticks is to soak them in water for a few hours ahead of time. So start your kabob prep early! Or use metal sticks, and be sure you don't forget your oven mitts.

Prep time: 10 minutes **Cook time:** 5 minutes
Makes: 6 servings

INGREDIENTS

1 pound jumbo shrimp, shelled and deveined
2 cloves garlic, finely chopped
2 tablespoons fresh parsley leaves, finely chopped
1 tablespoon fresh lemon juice
1/4 teaspoon sea salt
1/4 teaspoon freshly ground black pepper
2 green bell peppers, cut into 1-inch squares

1. Toss the shrimp, garlic, parsley, lemon juice, salt, and pepper in a large bowl until the shrimp are thoroughly coated. Set aside to marinate for 10 to 15 minutes. Meanwhile, heat the grill to medium-high.

2. Load up your kabob skewers, alternating the shrimp and bell peppers.

3. Grill the kabobs until the peppers have a light char and the shrimp is no longer translucent but is bright pink, approximately 2 minutes per side. Be careful not to overcook.

4. Remove the kabobs from the grill and serve on the stick or off, depending on your preference.

Veggie Tempura

I discovered this is the only way my son will eat vegetables, which I totally get. Sure, it's frying, but it's also lots of vitamins and minerals. So get on this method if you're trying to trick a kid into eating vegetables, or if you just love tempura and are so sad to be missing it when you dine out.

Prep time: 15 minutes **Cook time:** 5 minutes per batch
Makes: 4 servings

INGREDIENTS

2 cups canola oil
6 cups rice flour
1 egg white
4 cups seltzer
2 zucchini, quartered
1 yellow squash, quartered
1 sweet potato, cut in rounds
1 (8-ounce) block firm tofu, cut in squares
Hot mustard, for dipping
Wheat-free tamari, for dipping

1. Heat the oil in a deep skillet or deep fryer over medium-high heat.

2. In a large bowl, whisk together the rice flour, egg white, and seltzer until completely smooth.

3. Working in batches, submerge the vegetables and tofu in the flour mixture, covering the vegetables completely before removing and transferring them to the hot oil. Don't crowd the skillet; you'll need to flip the vegetables halfway through. Cook evenly for 5 minutes, or until golden brown.

4. Remove the vegetables from the oil and drain on a paper towel–covered plate. Serve with hot mustard and wheat-free tamari.

BBQ Chicken Meatballs

Stick a fancy toothpick in anything, and you've got a bang-up appetizer. For the easiest preparation, use gluten-free BBQ sauce in a jar. On a big game day or movie night, these are crowd pleasers. I think I might have eaten eight in one sitting, so mind yourself if you have company and try hard to share.

Prep time: 15 minutes **Cook time:** 25 minutes
Makes: 8 servings

INGREDIENTS

1 pound ground chicken
3 tablespoons gluten-free bread crumbs
1 egg, lightly beaten
1 teaspoon sea salt
1 teaspoon freshly ground black pepper
2 cups gluten-free BBQ sauce plus ½ cup for serving

1. Preheat the oven to 400°F.

2. In a large bowl, combine the ground chicken, bread crumbs, egg, salt, and pepper. Mix well, using your hands if you want.

3. Form the mixture into small balls approximately 1 inch in diameter and place on a shallow, lipped dish.

4. Pour 2 cups of the BBQ sauce over the meatballs and let them marinate for at least 10 minutes.

5. Place the meatballs on a greased baking sheet and bake for 25 minutes.

6. Remove the meatballs from the oven and serve with the remaining ½ cup BBQ sauce.

Sweet Potato Gnocchi

My brother sent me this recipe because he went Paleo for like, one week. Still, it's awesome, and now I feel fancy because I can make gnocchi! The trick with sweet potato gnocchi is to watch while you're mixing in your dry ingredients. Some sweet potatoes have more moisture than others and require more gluten-free flour. Others just need a little. I prefer my gnocchi with pesto, but you do you.

Prep time: 20 minutes **Cook time:** 1 hour plus 5 minutes per batch
Makes: 8 servings

INGREDIENTS

1 large sweet potato
1 cup all-purpose gluten-free flour, plus more if necessary
1 teaspoon baking soda
1 teaspoon sea salt
1 teaspoon white pepper
1 egg white
1 tablespoon butter

1. Preheat the oven to 450°F. Poke holes in the sweet potato, wrap it in foil, and bake it for 1 hour or until soft. Remove from the oven and allow to cool.

2. Remove the skin from the sweet potato and transfer the flesh to a medium bowl. Add the flour, baking soda, salt, and pepper and mix until smooth. Add more flour if the mixture is sticky.

3. Whisk the egg white until frothy and fold into the potato mixture. Cover in plastic wrap and refrigerate for at least 30 minutes.

4. Sprinkle flour on a large cutting board or a clean, even surface. Working with approximately one large handful of sweet potato dough at a time, roll dough between your hands to create a rope.

5. Place the ropes on the floured surface and, using a knife, cut each rope into pieces about 1 to 2 inches long. Use a fork's tines to indent the gnocchi with a line pattern across the dough.

6. Meanwhile, fill a large stockpot with water and bring to a boil. Working in batches, place 10 to 12 gnocchi in the boiling water. The gnocchi will float when they are done, after approximately 3 to 5 minutes. Drain well.

7. In a large skillet, melt the butter over medium-high heat. Transfer the cooked gnocchi to the skillet and cook for 2 to 3 minutes, tossing the gnocchi to coat evenly and get slightly crisp.

8. Serve the gnocchi with pesto (see recipe on page 139) or a gluten-free marinara sauce and Parmesan cheese.

. . . .

Paella

I realize this 100 percent shows my Cajun roots, but I like to think of paella as the Spanish version of jambalaya. Or maybe seafood risotto? Either way, it's super good and not nearly as difficult as one might think.

Oh, and I left out clams because I hate clams, but that is the traditional way to go. If you want to use them in this recipe, just add 8 to 10 clams to the skillet along with the shrimp.

Prep time: 25 minutes **Cook time:** 1 hour plus 1 hour marinating time
Makes: 10 servings

INGREDIENTS

3 pounds chicken thighs, bone in, skin on
1 teaspoon dried oregano
½ teaspoon red pepper flakes

½ teaspoon sea salt, plus more to taste
½ teaspoon freshly ground black pepper, plus more to taste
¼ cup olive oil
2 gluten-free chorizo sausages, sliced 1/4 inch thick
1 Spanish onion, diced
4 cloves garlic, crushed
1 bunch flat-leaf parsley, chopped, some reserved for garnish
1 (15-ounce) can whole tomatoes, drained and crushed by hand
3 cups short-grain Spanish rice
6 cups warm water
Generous pinch of saffron threads
1 pound jumbo shrimp, shelled and deveined
½ cup fresh sweet peas

1. Place the chicken thighs in a large dish and cover evenly with the oregano, red pepper, salt, and black pepper. Allow the chicken to marinate for at least 1 hour, refrigerated.

2. Heat the oil in a large, deep skillet (or paella pan if you have one) over medium-high heat for 1 to 2 minutes. Add the chorizo and cook for 3 to 4 minutes, stirring occasionally.

3. Place the chicken thighs in the pan skin-side down and cook until the skin is brown and slightly crispy, flipping after 5 to 7 minutes. Remove the sausage and chicken from the pan and set aside.

4. Add the onion, garlic, and parsley to the pan and cook for 2 to 3 minutes, until the onion and garlic start to soften. Add the tomatoes and cook for 5 minutes, until the sauce begins to thicken. Add the rice and stir to combine.

5. Add the water and turn the heat down to low, simmering for 10 to 15 minutes, stirring frequently, until the water begins to be absorbed.

6. Add the chicken and chorizo back to the pan along with the saffron. Simmer for 5 minutes, then add the shrimp. Simmer for 10 minutes more.

7. Turn the heat up to high for 45 seconds to crisp the rice. Add the peas, give the mixture a stir, and remove it from the heat.

8. Serve garnished with the reserved parsley.

. . . .

Chicken Pad Thai

I love a good pad thai, but sadly, either soy sauce or noodles usually contaminate it. But there are a few brands of gluten-free brown rice noodles you can use for this dish, so scoop them up and make pad thai whenever you're craving take-out. Substitute tofu for chicken breasts if you're leaning vegetarian.

Prep time: 15 minutes **Cook time:** 25 minutes
Makes: 4 servings

INGREDIENTS

8 ounces gluten-free brown rice noodles
4 tablespoons vegetable oil
2 cloves garlic, finely chopped
2 shallots, finely chopped
2 boneless skinless chicken breasts, cut into 1-inch cubes
4 tablespoons fresh lemon juice
3 tablespoons fish sauce
3 tablespoons sugar
½ teaspoon red pepper flakes
1 egg, lightly beaten
1 cup bean sprouts
4 tablespoons roasted peanuts
Cilantro (optional)
Lime wedges, for garnish

1. Cook the rice noodles according to the package directions. Drain and set aside.

2. In a large skillet, heat the oil over high heat for 1 minute, then turn the heat down to medium. Add the garlic and shallots and cook for 1 to 2 minutes. Add the chicken and cook, turning occasionally, for 10 minutes or until it is cooked through.

3. While the chicken is cooking, make the sauce: In a small bowl, whisk the lemon juice, fish sauce, sugar, and red pepper flakes together until the sugar is completely dissolved. Set aside.

4. Once the chicken is cooked, add the beaten egg to the skillet and scramble it with the chicken. Turn the heat down to low, add the cooked noodles, and stir to combine. Add the bean sprouts and peanuts and sauté for 1 minute. Pour in the sauce and cook for 1 minute more.

5. Serve with cilantro (if desired) and lime wedges.

· ·

Carrot Cake

I'm such a fan of bad-for-you foods that I usually won't eat carrot cake. I mean, vegetables? In cake? Who thought this was a good idea? In the case of this recipe, however, it's a dang good one. I brought this into my office and everyone flipped out. The applesauce makes it nice and moist and the icing, well, kills it. The cake was gone in 1.5 minutes. Srsly.

Prep time: 20 minutes **Cook time:** 35 minutes plus 2 hour rest time
Makes: 12 servings

INGREDIENTS

For the Cake:
2 cups all-purpose gluten-free flour, plus more for pans
2 teaspoons baking soda
1/2 teaspoon salt
2 teaspoons cinnamon
3 eggs
2 cups sugar
3/4 cup canola oil
3/4 cup buttermilk
2 teaspoons vanilla extract
2 cups grated carrot
1 cup applesauce
3/4 cup flaked coconut
1 cup chopped pecans, toasted

For the Frosting:
2 (8-ounce) packages cream cheese, softened
6 tablespoons butter, softened
1 1/2 teaspoons vanilla extract
5 cups confectioners' sugar, sifted
1 cup pecan pieces, toasted

1. Make the cake: Preheat the oven to 350°F. Grease and flour two 9-inch cake rounds.

2. In a small bowl, combine the flour, baking soda, salt, and cinnamon.

3. In a medium bowl, using a hand mixer, beat the eggs until fluffy. Add the sugar, oil, buttermilk, and vanilla and mix on medium speed.

4. Add the flour mixture and beat until combined.

5. Using a spoon or spatula, fold in the carrots, applesauce, coconut, and pecans. Pour the batter into the prepared cake pans and bake for 35 minutes, or until a toothpick inserted in the cake comes out clean. Remove the cake from the pans and transfer to a wire rack to cool.

6. Make the frosting: In a medium bowl, beat the cream cheese and butter until smooth and fluffy.

7. Add the confectioners' sugar 1 cup at a time, beating until completely combined between additions. Add the vanilla and mix well. Transfer to the refrigerator and allow to chill for 1 to 2 hours.

8. Assemble the cake: When the layers are cool and the frosting has chilled, frost the top of the first cake, then center the other cake on top and frost the top of that cake as well. Frost the sides and cover the sides with the pecans. Slice and serve.

· ·

Berry Crumble Pie

My grandmother made this pie with apples, but I prefer berry, well, anything. And I grab one of those frozen pie crusts or use a mix because I cannot deal. Please do that as well, because I want you to take it easy.

Prep time: 10 minutes **Cook time:** 55 minutes
Makes: 8 servings

INGREDIENTS

1 premade gluten-free piecrust
5 cups mixed berries (I prefer raspberries and blueberries)
2 tablespoons sugar
2 tablespoons fresh lemon juice
½ teaspoon cinnamon
½ cup brown sugar
½ cup all-purpose gluten-free flour

2 tablespoons cold butter
½ cup chopped pecans
Vanilla ice cream, for serving

1. Preheat the oven to 350°F. Bake the piecrust for 10 minutes, remove from the oven, and allow to cool.

2. Fill the cooled piecrust with the berries.

3. Combine the sugar, lemon juice, and cinnamon in a small bowl, then pour over the berries.

4. Combine the brown sugar and flour in a small bowl. Cut in the butter. Add the pecans and mix well. Sprinkle the mixture over the berries.

5. Bake for 45 minutes, or until the crumble topping is golden.

6. Remove the pie from the oven and allow it to cool for 5 to 10 minutes. Slice and serve with ice cream, or on its own.

. . . .

Ding Dong

Yep, I'm going there. While no one would argue Ding Dongs—gluten-free or not—are "healthy," I'd like to think that using no preservatives or chemicals in this version means we're eating a little bit healthier. Oh, who am I kidding? I just really think we deserve Ding Dongs.

Use the recipe for Jack's Devil's Food Cake (page 93; or hey, use a gluten-free devil's food cake mix if you're feeling tired) to make these.

Prep time: 20 minutes **Cook time:** 1 hour
Makes: 12 servings

INGREDIENTS

For the Cake:
Jack's Devil's Food Cake (page 93)

For the Fluffy Frosting:
⅓ cup whipping cream
1 tablespoon confectioners' sugar
½ teaspoon vanilla extract

For the Chocolate Ganache:
1 cup heavy cream
9 ounces semisweet chocolate, roughly chopped
  (or use semisweet chocolate chips)
1 tablespoon unsalted butter, at room temperature

1. Make the cake: Follow the instructions on page 94.

2. Make the frosting: Beat the cream and confectioners' sugar with an electric mixer until fluffy. Stir in the vanilla.

3. After the cake has cooled, turn it out onto a flat surface or large cutting board. Using a large, round cookie cutter, cut out approximately 12 (4½-inch) rounds and set them on a flat tray.

4. Using a sharp paring knife, remove a "button" ¾ inch in diameter from the center top of each cake, cutting halfway into the cake. Set each button aside; you will need them later.

5. Fill a pastry bag or zip-tight plastic bag with frosting. If using a zip-tight bag, cut the very tip off one corner so it can be used as a piping bag.

6. Fill the hole in each cake with frosting. Place each "button" back on top to cover the hole.

7. Make the ganache: Heat the cream over medium-high heat until simmering.

8. Place the chocolate in a medium bowl, then pour the hot cream on top. Allow the mixture to stand until the chocolate is mostly melted, 1 to 2 minutes.

9. Stir the butter into the chocolate mixture until smooth. Allow the chocolate ganache to cool for 5 to 10 minutes, then pour over each cake, smoothing out with a knife or spatula.

· ·

Campari et Pamplemousse

Let's finish these new recipes with a bang, shall we? I've recently discovered Campari and love it because I think all cocktails need a dash of color. Or a dash of alcohol.

Prep time: 2 minutes
Makes: 1 refreshing cocktail

INGREDIENTS

1 ounce Campari
2 ounces grapefruit juice
2 ounces club soda
Juice of ½ lime
1 lime wedge, for garnish

1. Pour the Campari and grapefruit juice over one large ice cube, or two smaller ice cubes, in a rocks glass. Stir.

2. Add the soda and lime juice and push on the ice gently to mix.

3. Serve with the lime wedge.

Resources

Where to eat, where to shop, and where to go when you need a shoulder to cry on—it's all here in my handy-dandy list, and *Gluten Is My Bitch* approved.

No, Really, You Can Eat Here

There are some restaurants that are so gluten-free friendly that you have to assume someone in the hierarchy is intimately acquainted with gluten poisoning. These places not only offer gluten-free options, but also understand that the preparation areas have to remain separate and go to great lengths to avoid cross-contamination. Some restaurants have sealed-off pizzas; others label every plate, bowl, and utensil to guarantee nothing goes awry. In contrast to simply offering a gluten-free menu, these places know how to serve it safely as well. Although it's true that the safety of every meal eaten outside your home depends upon all of those who prepare and serve it, you can feel safe at these joints that are paying strict attention.

Naturally, more restaurants are popping up right now that will do the gluten-free with no cross-contamination thing very well, but as of right now, these are the current stars of the genre. Some of these picks are local only in cities around the United States, and others are national. Visit each website to find a gluten-free location near you. As with every dining experience, call first to make sure they're ready for the gluten-free you.

All-Star Restaurants for the Gluten-Free

Big Bowl Chinese & Thai, bigbowl.com

Chuck E. Cheese's, (gluten-free pizza), chuckecheese.com

Fritzi Dog, fritzidog.com

Hugo's, hugosrestaurant.com

The Melting Pot, meltingpot.com

P.F. Chang's, pfchangs.com

Risotteria, risotteria.com

Ruby Foo's, rubyfoos.com

Story Tavern, storytavernburbank.com

Tula Gluten Free Bakery Cafe, tulabaking.com

2Good2B Bakery & Cafe, 2good2b.com

zpizza, zpizza.com

Bakeries

3 Fellers, 3fellersbakery.com

Babycakes NYC, babycakesnyc.com

Deerfields Bakery, deerfieldsbakery.com

Dempsey Bakery, dempseybakery.com

Everybody Eats, everybodyeats-inc.com

Flying Apron, flyingapron.com

Fonuts, fonuts.com

Kyra's Bake Shop, kyrasbakeshop.com

Mariposa Baking Company, mariposabaking.com

Rising Hearts Bakery, risingheartsbakery.com

Something Sweet Without Wheat, somethingsweetwithoutwheat.com

Sweet Freedom, sweetfreedombakery.com

Sweet 27, sweet27.com

Tu-Lu's Gluten-Free Bakery, tu-lusbakery.com

Whisk, whiskgfbakery.com

At the Store

If you're lucky, you'll find a ton of gluten-free options when you head to your local grocery. You can take them all home and have a crazy taste test, or you can try these delicious brands that my family picks again and again. Here are my favorite brands of prepackaged gluten-free goods.

Best Baking Mixes

Biscuits: Bob's Red Mill, Arrowhead Mills, Gluten Free Pantry

Cake/Cupcakes: XO Bakery: Kinnikinnick (Angel Food), Gluten Free Pantry, The Pure Pantry, Authentic Foods

Cornbread: Bob's Red Mill, Gluten Free Pantry

Pancakes: The Pure Pantry, XO Bakery, Arrowhead Mills

Piecrust: Gluten Free Pantry

Best Gluten-Free Pasta

Ancient Harvest Quinoa Pasta

Casalare

Mrs. Leeper's

RP's Pasta Company

Rustichella D'Abruzzo

Trader Joe's Corn Pasta

Best Gluten-Free Crackers

Blue Diamond

Crunchmaster Multi-Seed Crackers

Glutino Table Crackers

Skinny Crisps

Best Kid-Friendly Gluten-Free Food

Annie's Rice Noodle Mac & Cheese

Applegate GF Corn Dogs

Bell & Evans Chicken Tenders

Betty Crocker's Gluten-Free Cake Mix

Edward & Sons Gluten-Free Ice Cream Cones

Kinnikinnick graham crackers

Kinnikinnick K-Toos chocolate cookies

Best Gluten-Free Vitamins

Country Life Vitamins

Best Deli Meats

Applegate, Boar's Head

In the Kitchen

There are certain kitchen basics that every household needs, then there are some extra-special items that you're going to want in order to do some gluten-free baking, frying, and other amazing things. Additionally, if you still allow gluten in your house, you must have a dedicated pot(s), colander, utensils, and plates or bowls that are for gluten only. Never, ever touch those with your gluten-free food. Here's a basic list of kitchen tools because you're going to be spending a lot more quality time with your stove.

Necessary Tools in the Gluten-Free Kitchen

Liquid and solid measuring cups	Freezer-safe plastic containers	Cookie sheets (two)
Measuring spoons	Spatulas (two)	Square cake pan
Cutting boards (two)	Soup ladle	Round cake pans (two)
Large mixing spoons	Slotted spoon	Casserole dish
Whisk	Colander	Loaf pan
Set of knives (paring, bread, chef's)	Saucepans (two)	Deep fryer
	Frying pans (two)	Cuisinart Ice Cream Maker
Vegetable peeler	Roasting pan	Hand mixer
Cheese grater	Muffin tins (two)	Dutch oven
		Slow cooker

Where to Buy Gluten-Free Goods

Amazon, amazon.com	G-Free NYC, g-freenyc.com	Whole Foods, wholefoodsmarket.com
Better Batter, betterbatter.org	Swanson Health Products, swansonvitamins.com	Williams-Sonoma (Cup4Cup), williams-sonoma.com
Bob's Red Mill, bobsredmill.com	Vitacost, vitacost.com	

Gluten-Free Toys & Art Supplies for Kids

Discount School Supply offers an allergen listing for all of the school supplies it sells. Go to discountschoolsupply.com and search for gluten-free paints, clay, markers, and anything else Junior will put in his mouth.

Support Groups

Find your local chapter by checking out these national celiac organizations: **Celiac Disease Foundation** (celiac.org), **Celiac Support Association**, (csaceliacs.info), **National Foundation for Celiac Awareness** (celiaccentral.org)

Summer Camps for Celiac Kids

Camp Celiac—Rhode Island, campceliac.org
CDF Camp Gluten-Free—California, celiac.org

Paris Resources

Gluten-Free Groceries

La Vie Claire
(various locations), lavieclaire.com

Naturalia
(various locations), naturalia.fr

Farmers' Markets

Marché Bastille
Sundays only
Boulevard Richard-Lenoir
Paris, 11th Arrondissement

Saxe-Breteuil
Thursday, Saturday only
Avenue de Saxe
Paris, 7th Arrondissement

There are hundreds of markets—many available in the mornings on weekdays—throughout Paris. For a full listing, go to marches.equipements.paris.fr.

Gluten-Free-Friendly Restaurants

Le Coq Rico
98 Rue Lepic
Paris, 75018

Fée Nature
69 Rue d'Argout
Paris, 75002

Helmut Newcake
36 Rue Bichat
Paris, France (10th)
Telephone: +33 09 82 59 00 39

SOYA
20 Rue de la Pierre Lift
Paris 75011
Telephone: +33 01 48 06 33 02

West Country Girl
7 Passage Saint-Ambroise
Paris, 75011
westcountrygirl.com

Check out these blogs before you land in Paris:

David Lebovitz is an amazing writer and foodie. An American in Paris, he pretty much knows what we all want. Not gluten-free, but filled with delicious tips. davidlebovitz.com

Paris by Mouth is not only a great food blog with macaron round-ups, but it has a handy chart to tell you what is and what is not closed during those vacation months. parisbymouth.com

Acknowledgments

As with most gigantic projects like climbing Mount Everest or writing a funny book about gluten, there are many people who helped make this happen. This is where I thank those people. And yes, I did just compare sitting on my ass and writing this book with climbing Mount Everest.

Jennifer Levesque at Abrams for totally getting me in like five seconds, and Alison Fargis at Stonesong for the awesome agenting. That's why this book is here, you guys! Also the whole Stewart, Tabori & Chang/ABRAMS crew who escorted this book from the computer to the shelf.

Without the fantastically dressed and incredibly intelligent Dr. Ari Nowain, I would still be crapping my pants and wondering if it was the dairy. Thanks, Doc, for the quick diagnosis and patience for all of my questions.

Shazi Shabatian, my incredible nutritionist, for saying, "I can't wait to see your book," when I cried in her office that I couldn't possibly stop eating gluten because I'm a food writer. Also, for the fact checking and stellar information.

The incredible brain of Larry Smarr and his willingness to educate a layperson who is really just trying to get a laugh. Dr. Leah Klapper of BioLineRX who did the same.

Alicia Woodward of Living Without magazine, for not only fantastic information but also empathy and advice for a frustrated celiac.

Better Batter for providing me with testing materials, and Frank restaurant in Austin for keeping me in gluten-free beer and hot dogs.

Huge thanks to all of my loyal readers over at the www. Without you, well, I'd just be some irritated celiac writing a diary. Thank you for hating gluten as much as I do.

Rebecca Coleman for being cool and so connected that I'm pretty sure she can get me elected president of the United States of America.

To my lovely ladies, Victoria Harmer and Cary Fagan, who became determined to teach me how to cook more than chicken-fried steak, presumably because they were tired of hosting all of the dinner parties that did not utilize a deep-fat fryer.

Catherine Crawford for general radness, smartness, and dealing with me in times of hysteria.

My Paris advisory committee: Anna Clark Muntz, Jessica Lee-Rami, Stéphane Zuccolotto, and the Goldmans of the Northwest.

Basic awesomeness and attractiveness with the occasional taste testing: Mac Montandan, Ada Calhoun, Gwynne Watkins, Amy Boshnack, Kara Dean & The Assael Dudes, Soleil Moon-Frye, Nancy Dillon, Rob Anderson, Laurie Kilmartin, Bart Coleman, Kiran and Joby Mahto, Caroline Donahue, Geoff Peveto, Dad, Lorieann, Nicole Mensinger, Abe Bradshaw, and ELI.

The Peveto/Reeves contingency have offered recipes, support, and autoimmune diseases by the bucketful. Thank you so much for most of that. The Goldmans have allowed a shiksa to deep-fry pork for them with nary a complaint. Especially Amy and Ellen, who have provided me with so many gluten-free pies and cakes to enjoy.

And last but never, ever, ever least—my beautiful family. Aaron Goldman has offered support beyond that of a normal human husband and makes encourages me to finish what I start. Esmé and Judah helped put my life into laser focus and consistently crack me the hell up. You guys are the most amazing people in the entire universe. Period.

Conversion Charts

Weight Equivalents

AVOIRDUPOIS	METRIC
¼ oz	7 g
½ oz	15 g
1 oz	30 g
2 oz	60 g
3 oz	90 g
4 oz	115 g
5 oz	150 g
6 oz	175 g
7 oz	200 g
8 oz (½ lb)	225 g
9 oz	250 g
10 oz	300 g
11 oz	325 g
12 oz	350 g
13 oz	375 g
14 oz	400 g
15 oz	425 g
16 oz (1 lb)	450 g
1 ½ lb	750 g
2 lb	900 g
2 ¼ lb	1 kg
3 lb	1.4 kg
4 lb	1.8 kg

Volume Equivalents

AMERICAN	METRIC	IMPERIAL
1/4 tsp	1.2 ml	
1/2 tsp	2.5 ml	
1 tsp	5.0 ml	
1/2 Tbsp (1.5 tsp)	7.5 ml	
1 Tbsp (3 tsp)	15 ml	
1/4 cup (4 Tbsp)	60 ml	2 fl oz
1/3 cup (5 Tbsp)	75 ml	2.5 fl oz
1/2 cup (8 Tbsp)	125 ml	4 fl oz
2/3 cup (10 Tbsp)	150 ml	5 fl oz
3/4 cup (12 Tbsp)	175 ml	6 fl oz
1 cup (16 Tbsp)	250 ml	8 fl oz
1 1/4 cups	300 ml	10 fl oz (1/2 pint)
1 1/2 cups	350 ml	12 fl oz
2 cups (1 pint)	500 ml	16 fl oz
2 1/2 cups	625 ml	20 fl oz (1 pint)
1 quart	1 liter	32 fl oz

Oven Temp Equivalents

OVEN MARK	F	C	GAS
very cool	250-275	130-140	1/2-1
cool	300	150	2
warm	325	170	3
moderate	350	180	4
moderately hot	375-400	190-200	5-6
hot	425-450	220-230	7-8
very hot	475	250	9

INDEX